HAYAGREEVA

The Guru of Goddess Saraswati

Discover some lesser known facts about Hayagreeva and Saraswati and her journey in Svarga Loka and Bhu Loka

Saraswati Raman

Inquiries and Book Orders should be addressed to:

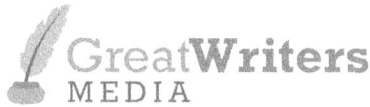

Great Writers Media
Email: info@greatwritersmedia.com
Phone: 877-600-5469

ISBN: 978-1-960605-45-0 (sc)
ISBN: 978-1-960605-46-7 (ebk)

CONTENTS

INTRODUCTION

Lord Vasudeva, from his abode in Shri Vaikuntha himself incarnated as Shri Hayagreeva on this Earth. Singing his praise is sufficient to vanish all troubles like the Sun whose rays at dawn are sufficient to dispel all darkness of the night.

It is believed that worship of Shri Hayagreeva can bestow upon the devotee the divine vision to know the events of the future. He taught the Vedas to Brahmadeva and Lalita Sahasranamam to Agastya Muni. Anyone who surrenders at his holy feet will be blessed with the good fortune of not only enjoying all prosperity here but also attains the abode of Shri Narayana.

In my exploration on the Alwars and Goddess Saraswati I had come across a lot of information about Shri Hayagreeva. I decided to put them altogether in the form of a book.

I had been acquainted with Shri Hayagreeva as the deity for education and intellectual achievements.

I express my deep sense of gratitude to Shri Raghottaman Babu and Smt. Uma Babu for extending their assistance in several ways during the times of writing this book. I whole heartedly pray that Shri Hayagreeva bless them with all prosperity and happiness.

Shri Hayagreeva showers his knowledge on all students and so also is Goddess Saraswati who blesses each one with learning and is worshipped the world over. If one like her could remove her jingling anklet for the sake of hearing the songs of Andadi, is it not an indication of the heights of her command over the Tamil language? I have compiled tastefully, the information about the Goddess and the songs written in her praise by poets who have been blessed with her Grace alone, in this volume. All the readers of this book will definitely receive the blessings of Shri Hayagreeva and the Goddess of Arts and learning, of which I have not the least doubt whatsoever.

The four armed Goddess, is seen holding the conch and the holy beads in her two hands on the back and showing the Mudra of granting blessing and a book in the hands in front.

She is seated on a bright white lotus shining like the exposed portion of a sphatik stone. A blemishless body with a horse face is Shri Hayagreeva who is the God for learning. May His benevolent gaze forever shine upon me.

1

Characteristic features
of Shri Hayagreeva

I f there was someone who could be a teacher to Goddess Saraswati herself, it was Shri Hayagreeva. He had actually manifested before one of the Vaishnava Acharyas, Shri Vedanta Desikar and blessed him with the spit from his mouth. After that the poetic ability of Desikar expanded exponentially. Besides he even excelled in all the sixty four arts as a result of which he was felicitated with the title of Sarva Tantra Swatantra by Mother Goddess Ranganayaki of Tiruvaranganatha temple herself.

Hayagreeva was always seen in a brilliant white color, sparkling white neck like a sphatik, a strong and sturdy body, eyes brimming with knowledge, whose glory has been sung in scriptures like the Mahabharata, Devi Bhagavat and Hayagreeva Kalpa.

During the period of Ramayana, it is said that Hanuman, in order to gain additional strength for lifting the Sanjeevani Mountain, had prayed to the idol of Hayagreeva.

Guru Muni Agastya is said to have had the darshan of Shri Hayagreeva himself while he was doing penance at Kancheepuram and had personally instructed him.

The vision that Swami Desikar had of Shri Hayagreeva in a globular light at Tiruvayindipur was etched out and can still be seen there.

Hayagreeva's manifestation can be seen not only in the Indian culture and the Hindu traditions but also in several other parts of the world as well in some form or the other. An instance of this is the Buddhist religion, where a mention of him appears in several places.

Since he neighed like a horse and drove off enemies encountered, Tibetans who are horse traders worship Hayagreeva as their Deity for Protection and a book containing the rituals for this worship has also been published. Besides, they also believe in the existence of a 108 Hayagreevas who take care of human beings and animals in treating skin diseases. More particularly for diseases like leprosy in human beings, the Tibetans believe him to cure them.

In Japan and Tibet, we can see among the Buddhists the practice of worship of horse faced gods, which occupies a pride of place in their rituals. This has been attributed to a sacred disciple, Ayaksha of the Buddhist monk Avalokideeshwara. You can notice this even in the similarity of the sounds of the names Hayagreeva and Ayaksha.

Besides, in the Vedas there is a mention of Hayagreeva as two separate Gods. This has been adopted as a fact by the Buddhist religion. One of the gods was considered by the early Buddhists as the Lord who causes obstacles while the other was considered among the Vajrayana Buddhists to be the God who bestowed knowledge.

Tibetan religious texts address Hayagreeva as Dharmapal. He is believed to have incarnated in those lands for bestowing upon the people the knowledge of all the arts. The skin diseases of man are said to be passed on from the snake species as a form of punishment. The uniqueness of Dharmapal was his ability to treat and cure incurable diseases in man, more particularly the skin diseases. Even terminal diseases like leprosy is said to have been cured under his hands as described in those books.

The Japanese Mahayana Buddhist religion considers Avalokideeshwara to be one who looked after the horses. He is said to come riding on his horse and throw his benevolent glance over the horses tied in the stable. A depiction of this writing can also be seen as a sculpture in stone which has been found where Avalokideeshwara is seen riding on his horse. The vehicle on which he is seated appears to have the head of a horse and not that of Hayagreeva.

In this manner, Hayagreeva who appears to have occupied a pride of place in the culture of the people in different parts of the world, is also attributed with having sung and instructed the Lalita Sahasranamam. It is by chanting of this Stotra of Hayagreeva that Shri Vedanta Desikar and Shri Vadiraj had become the ocean of knowledge that they are well known for.

The Vaishnavas still believe that a portion of the Sanjeevani Mountain that Hanuman carried fell off and that is the present Tiruvahindrapuram. It was on this mountain that Shri Hayagreeva had given darshan to Shri Desikar. We shall come back to this story later in the book.

Go to Chettipunniyam

My friend's wife complained every time I met her about her daughter who was now appearing for the plus 2 exams. Although she didn't appear to show much interest in her studies, she agreed to study hard whenever she was questioned about it.

My wife rejoined her saying that some children were like that and suggested as to why not take her to Cheetti Punniyam and make her have the darshan of Hayagreeva at the temple there.

Presently, the name of Chettipunniyam attains prominence during the approach of school and college exams, in and around the region of Chennai. What is so special about the place?

It is here that Shri Hayagreeva, the God for knowledge and learning is said to have manifested.

The importance of education cannot be overemphasized in today's competitive world. If there were no schools it is as though there was no education itself. Therefore it is important that children do well in their studies and parents too hope they get good marks in their exams. Besides, if one had to procure admission in any college, firstly, one has to have the money or else have good marks. Such is the situation. Therefore every parent goads his child and pushes him or her to study harder, literally beyond their limits.

In such circumstances it is natural for average students to fall short somewhere or the other. It is for this reason that parents want their children to somehow or the other get good marks and for this they go to any extent.

There are more things in this world to be known than known. This is what Tiruvalluvar highlighted when he said, "Arithorum Ariyamai Kandatral". When we go to study a subject, we then discover to our knowledge and surprise as to how much deeper we can delve into it and how much more intricate the details of it really are. There is also the anxiety and perplexing knowing that this had remain hidden to us all this while. This is the beauty of education.

Education can provide all the conveniences of life. It is considered essential as well. There may be challenges while learning. But will it give satisfaction? The answer is no.

Can you give an example of this?

Definitely so! Some men and women who earn ten lakhs and fifteen lakh packages in some of the corporate companies today, not satisfied with the work or the work pressures involved are seen to even commit suicide as reported in the newspapers these days.

As far as we are concerned, isn't ten lakhs a year a sufficient sum of money to get us through? "Your father had not even earned two lakh rupees a year" is what some women try to convince their children. But they are not in a position to accept that. The reason being their needs have outgrown and along with it the desires of the mind as well.

Conveniences can end. It is the mental satisfaction that provides stability and joy. This is the reason why knowingly or unknowingly we all crave for joy. We begin to understand the need for an education that provides joy over an education that provides temporary happiness.

The joy of Brahma is considered to be Eternal bliss or Brahmananda. The crest jewel holding this bliss like the blemishless sphatik stone in the form of absolute pure ocean of knowledge is Shri Hayagreeva. He is the guru for all kinds of learning. Besides he is also the Guru to the Goddess Saraswati who provides us the skills for the sixty four types of arts.

Education and knowledge

The bridge among the Vaishnavites and Shaaktas is Shri Hayagreeva. It was he who taught the Sri Lalita Sahasranamam to Agastya Muni and who took it to the pinnacle of glory accepted by the worshippers of Sri Vidya. He is the Lord of education and knowledge. Some may ask, "Is education and knowledge different from each other?"

Reading books and the understanding that we get from them is called information. This is limited. It is set to boundaries. For example, those who have graduated in Engineering may not know anything about medicine. Similarly those who are experts in cooking cannot do accounts. But knowledge is not like that. It is all encompassing. It is like the sky. That, knowing which, everything else is known that is understood as Brahma.

If one attains this knowledge then he needs nothing else. That is why the great poet Bharati questioned, "If I get this knowledge what need have I for anything else?"

The Upanishads reiterate that knowledge knowing which nothing else need to be known is called Brahma. In order to have the knowledge of that Brahma one has to have the knowledge of Maya. One who showers this knowledge and one who is the authority over this is the Lord with the face of a horse. Shri Hayagreeva had the face of a horse. Hence the ancient Tamil addressed him as Parimukha Deva. Pari means horse in Tamil.

Knowledge and education are like the two eyes to man. Blessing him with these two things, Shri Hayagreeva makes his life enlightened. Those who have education are like people who have eyes but no vision. Therefore it is essential that we worship this God who showers us with knowledge. He is no ordinary Guru. He is the guru to Goddess Saraswati herself, the embodiment of all arts.

About 3 kms away from the Shri Hayagreeva temple at Chettipunniyam in Chennai is the Narasimha temple which can be reached from Tambaram by bus (60 C) which goes via Chettipunniyam. It is open for darshan from 7:30 in the morning to 12 in the afternoon and reopens from 4:30 to 8 pm. Do visit and gain the blessings.

2

The horse faced Lord who gives knowledge

Importance of Education

Our body may be destroyed on death, but that which accompanies us through all our lifetimes is knowledge. Therefore we should devote a major portion of our time and energy to gain that knowledge through education.

Education cannot be destroyed through water. It cannot be burnt in fire. Thieves cannot steal it. It will only grow by sharing it with others but will not diminish. Not much effort is required in shielding it. When education has so many advantages, should we not try to gain it somehow or the other?

Tiruvalluvar writes:

Yaadaanum Naadaamal Uraamal Yennoruvan Shantunaiyum Kallada Vaaru.

Education does not have banks like the river. In our limited lifetime, a little knowledge goes a long way in relieving us of several kinds of diseases that dog mankind, while a good education is capable of making it beautiful, plentiful and prosperous. Then alone man's birth as a human being gets complete fulfillment. He becomes a man not by body alone but by a higher attributes of living as well.

It is for this reason that education is given a high pedestal in importance in all literature, history books and Puranas.

"Educating young is like etching on stone" is an old saying. The education that we get at a young age gets etched in our minds like that on stone. That is our guide for our future and that becomes our foundation for all decisive choices that we make in our life. If the foundation is strong then the building that stands upon it will last strongly for several years into the future. If we are to lead a healthy life then we should feed our children with good education very early in life.

The great Tiruvalluvar writes that the educated alone are human beings and all those who are not educated are equivalent to animals. Therefore, we who have known the importance of education so much have shown inextinguishable thirst for Eternal knowledge.

Those amongst us who toil day in and day out to accumulate material things which are subject to destruction and impermanent, should devote more time and energy in understanding the importance of assimilation through education and then exert in attaining it systematically.

Students who persevere in this manner, those engaged in colleges, teachers, those who yearn for higher education are bound to face some problem or the other in course of time. There is a possibility that one may fail to succeed serially in the desired course of higher education. This is bound to make one depressed.

One may yearn for that singular opportunity at what we dream of. Perhaps we may chance upon it after years of waiting. But the chance of enjoying it may be grabbed away by some other person. Such failures, sorrows, are unavoidable. If we are to overcome them, or avoid them crossing our path, we have to pray to Shri Hayagreeva.

Go on exile to the forest

Let us look into an incident from the Ramayana.

Rama was to be coroneted in the morning and the date and day had been decided by Sage Vasishtha after astrological calculations.

Chakravarthi Dasharatha was enthusiastically waiting to see Rama crowned the King. But did everything go as pre-planned? It didn't go, right?

On the morning of the coronation, Sumantra, Dasharatha's Minister came looking for Rama as Kaikeyi had called for him. When he met Kaikeyi, he found his father Dasharatha lying unconscious in her quarters.

Not understanding the situation, Rama looks at Kaikeyi for an answer. Looking at Rama, she says, "The King is in no condition to speak now. On an earlier occasion, he had granted me two boons which I asked him to fulfill now. He too agreed to it. That is why he has become so sad."

"As per my demanded boons, you have to go to the forest for fourteen years and spend your time there as a monk. The position of King assigned to you will now be handed over to my son Bharat. Not having the courage to tell you this has made your father sorrowful. Accepting the King's command gracefully go to the forest; until then I shall not eat the royal food nor wear royal clothes." She tells him solemnly.

The Kingdom which was to go to Rama was in an instant stolen away.

Was it the cheating of Mantara the maid? Or was it Rama's destiny is another matter altogether.

The Tapping Tantrics

There have been several such stories of stealing away the food in hand before it even reaches the mouth not only in the ancient times but even in the contemporary period as narrated in the collection of stories in a book by the grandfather of Tamil, Uvesa in his book, The Periya Tirukkundram Subbarama Iyer.

Among the very famous doyens of music in Tamil Nadu, Shri Tirukkundram Subbarama Iyer, occupies an important place. He is proficient not only in singing but also in reciting Tamil poems.

Even though there have been many artists and whistlers in our country, their works and special acts have been lost into oblivion with the passage of time. The main reason for this is that they have written them in the context of the political leadership prevailing during their times. Those who sing in praise of the Lord have become immortal even after death.

Hundreds of scholars have penned thousands of literary works in Tamil Nadu. Many of them have been lost. The reason for that is that instead of offering their talent to God, they sang in expectation of monetary benefits.

Subbarama Iyer, instead of making this mistake, persisted in making his compositions in singing the praise of the Lord. The devotion filled in his heart for the Lord expressed itself through his songs.

Subbarama Iyer's songs had the depth worthy of inclusion amongst the works of Tanjavur literary empire of scholars. Having lived in Tanjavur itself during the reign of Sarbhoji, he had the occasion to come face to face with the King several times and exhibit his unique talent.

After Sarbhoji, Shivaji came to rule. He did not get the opportunity to come as close to Shivaji, as he could to his father Sarbhoji. Yet, being a familiar place and also considering the Empire to be a worthy place to be in, he continued to live there.

Around that time, Shivakozundhu Desikar of Kottayur created a play titled Kuruvanchi. It got wide acclaims. So, everyone persuaded Subbarama Iyer too to create a play on Shivaji on the line of Kuruvanji.

To him, who had attained proficiency in literary works, this was not an impossible task. Hence within a short time, he created a Kuruvanchi. But for some reason it did not gain any popularity. Even praise from the critics was not to that extent.

After that, at the request of some officials, Subbarama Iyer composed five Ragas on Emperor Shivaji in the form of five Kirtanam compositions. Those who heard listened to those Kirtanais were all in praise of Subbarama Iyer. Even Emperor Shivaji was appreciative of them after listening to them and was overjoyed. Expressing his joy he presented Subbarama Iyer with a village as a token of his appreciation.

Jealous about this, some people started instigating the Emperor. They said, that the Maharaja should not listen to Tamil songs. They frightened him saying that "If he did his lineage itself would be destroyed." The Maharaja who had already lost his freedom and luxuries coming under the influence of the British, was further frightened by these instigations and without much investigation believed them.

He pondered over the fact that bad luck was already dogging his footsteps and as if that were not enough, if these Kirtanais would further torment him, then what could be worse than that, he thought.

If he had true and heartfelt regard towards Tamil and Tamil literary scholars and musicians, then he would have ignored the taunting of these jealous people. It is said that all things dark appear to be ghosts to a defeated King. Considering the precarious circumstances prevailing then around the King, it is understandable that the King had begun to doubt and hesitate over everything he came across.

Subbarama Iyer came to know of the gift of appreciation given by Emperor Shivaji and also the instigations by the jealous persons that had resulting in the King being prejudiced against him.

He did not regret the loss of land that was to be his own. Realizing that continuing to remain in such a place would only bring harm and loss to him and to the Tamil language, he left for his native place.

These incidents only go to reveal how the world of art and artists whom the world showers with praise and accolades too have to face such unavoidable setbacks when those in power shy away in face of difficulties.

Whatever the fate, it can be saying enough is enough, is it not?

For such people Shri Hayagreeva's blessings can come to the rescue and the obstacles can be averted. Where we have his blessings, we can boldly sing, "what can time do? What can obstacles do? What can serious allegations do?" His grace will bring his blessings to us without any obstructions.

He will give us the wealth for education

He is praised and worshipped as the God of Knowledge for having brought back the Vedas that were stolen and hidden by the Asuras in the Patala Loka. Worshipping him brings all skills within one's command. This is not ordinary education. It is a wealth bestowing education. In the modern times, is it sufficient to have only education? One should be able to earn a living out of that. Is it not? Should we not have an education that ensures that?

We see many parents grumbling that, "My son studied well, he got a degree, but could not get a good job." If such a situation is to be avoided, they should surrender at the feet of Shri Hayagreeva.

As the God of Education he will bless you with a rewarding education. The reason being, he is the Lord of Education. Granting darshan along with Shri Hayagreeva is Sri Laxmi Devi. Therefore worshipping them whole heartedly will ensure no shortfall in wealth and knowledge.

A horse while galloping towards its goal, does not look this side or that side. It focuses all its energy and efforts on one point and attains its goals. For students also, while pursuing their education, Shri Hayagreeva will help in keeping their attention concentrated on their studies so as to maximize the results.

3

Incarnation of Hayagreeva

How did he manifest? What was the reason for his manifestation? What is the background? Let us get to know about this presently.

At the time of the great deluge, eggs and living species lay drowned in the waters. The Supreme Lord, Paramatman, Shri Narayana was floating on a banyan leaf. After the lapse of a prolonged period of time, he had the desire to once again begin Creation. He manifested Brahma from the lotus of his naval. He also created the Vedas that would be of assistance in the process of creation of this world and presented him with them. Brahma, with the support of the Vedas created the world and all the creatures in it. In this manner the world of Creation began.

Once two drops of water emerged from the naval of the Paramatman and they manifested as two Asuras by the name of Madhu and Kaitabh. They considered themselves superior to Brahma himself. In order that this may be accepted by all, they decided to do some such disastrous thing that would make Brahma to bring all creation to a halt.

Doing good is difficult but doing evil is not that way. It can be easily accomplished, is it not? Both the Asuras assumed the form of two huge horses. Their target was not Brahma but the Vedas with the support of which Brahma was carrying out the work of Creation of the Universe.

Both of them set out and reached Satya Loka. They seized the Vedas from Brahma and returned to Patal Loka.

The writing plume for the writer, the hammer and nail to the sculptor when seized from their craftsmen would render them job-less, so also was the situation of Brahma when he was left without the Vedas. How was the work of creation to be carried on in the world? With this question looming large before him, Brahma went to the Deva Loka and approached the other Devas and explained his position to them. They too were helpless. All of them decided to go to Shri Narayana.

They prayed to him, "O Protector from difficulties! O Preserver of the Orphaned! The Asuras have taken away forcefully the Vedas that were the support for creation of the Universe. You alone can bring them back to us and help us carry on the work of Creation."

Madhava who had assumed several incarnations for fulfilling the requests of his devotees, now manifested as a horse for procuring the Vedas from the Asuras. Since the Asuras had seized the Vedas taking the form of horses, the Paramatman too decided to take the same form for retrieving the Vedas.

Hence he set off with the face of a horse, body of man and shining splendidly like a crore Suns. The form of Shri Hayagreeva had the Sun and the Moon as his eyes, and Ganga and Saraswati as the eyelids. In this Divine form the Lord went and killing Mdhu and Kaitabh, he procured the Vedas. This was the story of the incarnation of Shri Hayagreeva. There are different stories in the various Puranas related to this incarnation, one of which says that he incarnated as a Tortoise. We shall see that later on in the book.

Since they were chased by Asuras, the Vedas felt that they had become polluted and were aggrieved. So, the Lord with the horse's face snorted and with the whiff of air from his nostrils, he purified the Vedas.

After waging an intense battle with the Asuras, the anger in the form of Shri Hayagreeva did not cool down. Brahma, seeing him in that obsessed condition, took Mahalakshmi and brought her before him.

The Lord, on seeing her, was pacified and seating his beloved Goddess on his lap, he presented the darshan of Sri Lakshmi Hayagreeva.

Mahalakshmi in the body of a horse

The word Haya means horse. The Goddess with the face of a horse was Ashwaruda. She was born from the chord of Affection of the Goddess. She was a warrior who led an army of crores of horses on behalf of the Goddess on the battlefield.

There are specific vehicles for the temple of Shiva, and some other specific vehicles for the Vishnu temple. Shiva has the Nandi while Vishnu has the Garuda. Although there are such differences, the common vehicle for both the temples is the horse. The horse faced Hayagreeva has instructed the Devi Mahatmyam to Agastya Muni.

Ashwini Kumars have horse faces. Unable to bear the intense heat of the Sun, his wife Usha couldn't co-habit with him and so assumed the form of a horse and started dwelling in the forest. This was at the place where the two rivers, River Kalindi and River Tamasa converged. Mahalakshmi too arrived there in the form of a female horse.

Why did Mahalakshmi assume the form of a horse? That is an interesting story.

It was not an interesting story but the result of a curse that had befallen her. Mahalakshmi had manifested during the churning of the ocean of Milk. Along with her, a white horse too manifested, by the name of Ucchaisarivas. The horse was very beautiful and strong. There was not even a single black spot on its body. It was as white as the milk of the ocean from which it had emerged. It was fascinating to the eyes of all present there.

One day, Mahalakshmi happened to see Sun's son Ravi riding on that horse and proceeding towards Swarga Loka. The handsome white body of Ucchasravas held her gazing at it spell bound. Bound in the affection of his beloved, and observing her enjoying the beauty of the sight, Narayana happened to ask her as to who was it that was riding on the horse.

It was not the appropriate moment for such a question to Mahalakshmi. She ignored what her husband said to her and continued gazing at the horse and relishing the sight. Narayana was annoyed by her indifference to what he had asked.

"Did the horse become more important to her than me?" was the question that came up in his mind. He cursed her, "If that is so then be born on the Earth as a horse."

It was that horse that arrived there. After cursing Mahalakshmi to be born as a horse, Mahavishnu, became restless in the Milky ocean. He too took the form of a male horse and arrived there and pacifying her he became friendly with her. The son born out of the union was Ekvira.

Yayati's son Durvas did penance and procured this Ekvira as his son.

When Usha had taken the form of a female horse, Sun too took the form of a male horse and joined her. They gave birth to the Ashwini Kumars. This was how they had horse face. Due to Mahavishnu having assumed the form of a horse as well as his having assumed the face of a horse for killing Madhu and Kaitabh, the temples of Vishnu given prominence to the Horse as the vehicle of the Lord.

For the sake of Manicka Vasakar Lord Shiva made the foxes into horses and later he converted the horses into foxes and showed his Leela. At that time Nandi himself became a horse for him which is why even in Shiva Temples we have the horse as the vehicle for festivities.

The horse has several credits to it. A horse that is extremely strong is used for the worship of Ashwaruda. She herself worships the holy feet of the Goddess Mahalakshmi. How can one describe the glory of the Goddess herself?

There are separate rituals for the worship of the Goddess during the Ashvamedha yagna. To bring the whole world under one rule, the Chakravarti King conducts an Ashvamedha yagna in which a horse is sent to all the countries. Anyone who catches hold of the horse is understood to be ready for war. When Shri Rama had sent the Ashvamedha horse, Luv and Kush had caught hold of it. This incident however, instead of beginning a war ended on a peaceful note. It was because of this yagna that Shri Rama was able to identify his sons.

It is with this glorious heritage that the horse faced incarnation of Shri Hari as Shri Hayagreeva took place.

Ashvamedha Yagna horse

The emperors of the ancient times performed the Ashvamedha yagna with the same fervor and enthusiasm as the Rajasuya yagna and in a grand manner. Under this yagna, the King sent a horse with his banner tied to its face, decorating it in a grand manner with his victory flag and sent it to all the countries around his Kingdom.

Every King who welcomed the horse and showed their respects is said to have accepted the King as the Chakravarti. Anyone who opposed would capture the horse and tie it up. Immediately the King who sent the horse had to fight against the King who had tied up the horse and win over him. In this manner several countries were visited some of whom became his friends and resulted in establishing the fact that the King was worthy of conducting an Ashvamedha yagna.

At the end of the yagna, the flagship horse that was sent by the King was sacrificed. The horse selected for the Ashvamedha yagna could even be the one that has participated in several battles as well. As a result the moment it is brought into the Yagnashala it becomes purified considerably. For this purpose necessary purification mantras are chanted by the Vedic pundits.

Those mantras speak of its greatness. The Krishna Yajurveda Taittreya Samhita Yagna horse purification mantras are spread across several Slokas. Its four legs are described as representing the four Vedas, and is also indicative of the four directions. Its head indicates the East which represents the early morning, the eyes stand for the Sun, the breath of air stands for the one common air that flows through the five primordial elements. The birth of the Yagna horse is said to be from the ocean of Milk. Its glory is comparable to the Divine horse, Ucchaisiravas, and its purification and the mantra japa through which it is elevated is mentioned in the scripture.

Vishwarupa Darshan –the merit of the yagna

During the times of the Mahabharata, when Shri Krishna went as the messenger of the Pandavas from Hastinapur, Duryodhana had conceived a plan to kill him. At that time, apart from killing those who attacked him, he also rose to an enormous size to reveal his Vishwarupa darshan thereby re-establishing his glory.

Long after the Mahabharata war had ended, Rishi Vaishampayan was reporting about all that happened to King Janame Jayan. On that day he expressed his desire to have the glimpse of that Vishwarup darshan of Shri Krishna. He pleaded to Maharishi to tell him if there was a way for that.

The Maharishi replied a way for that and told the King that if he went to Satyavrata Kshetra Kanchipuram and conduct a Ashvamedha yagna there, then at the end of it, you will get your desired Shri Krishna's Vishwarupa Darshan and bless you.

The King also went to Kanchipuram and performed an Ashvamedha yagna on a grand scale as a result of which Shri Krishna appeared from the center of the yagna kund and gave his vishwarupa darshan. The King and Harita Muni were filled with joy on seeing this astonishing sight.

There is a temple built for Shri Krishna at Kancheepuram even today symbolic of the Vishwarupa darshan of Shri Krishna to the Pandavas. This is one of the 108 divine Vaishnava Kshetras. The main deity is seen giving darshan facing east. This is the biggest idol of Shri Krishna in any temple in the whole of India.

As the fruits of the Ashvamedha yagna, Jayameyajan got the Vishwarupa darshan of Shri Krishna. The Pandavas too had performed an Ashvamedha yagna. As the fruits thereof they received a very important instruction from the young one of a mongoose. Let us get to know about that incident as well.

4

A golden colored mongoose

After winning over the battle of Kurukshetra, and after taking over the reins of the Kingdom, one day Dharma felt uneasy, restless and lonely. What was the way to get rid of it? When he went and asked Bhagwan Vyasa about it, he advised to conduct an Ashvamedha yagna after which if he would feed the poor he would attain peace of mind.

Accordingly, Yudhishtir performed an Ashvamedha yagna on a very grand scale. All the Pandavas participated in it very enthusiastically. More than a hundred Vedic pundits chanted the mantras. Every day, thousands of people partook of the food and returned happily. No Chakravarti had every performed such a yagna and food distribution on such a large scale. The people spoke about it amongst each other.

The Pandavas were taken over with pride. They felt that there could be no chakravarthi worth the name like themselves. The arrogance of having conducted such an Ashvamedha yagna in such a grand manner was reflected in their speech.

One day, in front of everybody's sight, within the yagnashala, a mongoose entered hastily. One portion of its body was shining like gold. Everyone looked at that mongoose with curiosity. Ignoring everybody, it went straight up to a pile of edible flour and jumping on it started rolling in it.

What kind of a surprise was this? Expecting that the golden colored mongoose would enter the kitchen area and consume some of the food there, they were surprised that it did nothing of that sort but merely rolled on the flour that was placed there.

After having surprised them in this manner, it gave one more surprise to them. It looked at them and started speaking. It said, "Everyone is saying that this is a very big yagna. Believing them I came here. But I don't think this is anything big." Saying this it went to a corner and lay down. Seeing this sight, the Munis and the common people including the Kings were shocked and stood there spell bound and breathless.

Hearing this, Dharmaputra arrived there. Addressing the mongoose he asked angrily, "Who are you? What do you mean by finding faults with this yagna?"

The golden body of the mongoose moved just a bit slightly. Gazing with its reddish colored eyes intensely at him, it said, "if a person is performing a yagna for some gain, then it falls down in stature by a small extent. From the food distribution that you are doing here feeding thousands of people daily, have you been able to save any one of them at least from hunger? No. All those who eat here are all well to do people, are they not?"

"Besides, you are having all the means and wealth at your disposal. Therefore you are looking for fame by feeding so many people. Do you know how great it is for a family to feed another without anyone else knowing about it?" After elaborating in this manner, the mongoose looked at Dharmaputra and said, "Annadata Dharmaputra, listen to my story. Then alone will you be able to fully understand the situation completely." Saying thus, it went on to describe an incident.

"Some time earlier, I had been to the house of a poor family. They had no means for the next meal. The head of that family used to bring food home daily by begging and that too while chanting the Lord's names and wearing torn clothes. Besides he would go only to three streets. He would not stand in front of any house."

"As he went along chanting the names of the Lord and singing his bhajans, the ladies of the house respectfully would call out to him, ask him to wait and would offer food to him. In this manner he would collect food only from five houses. Beyond that, if anyone offered, he would refuse. He would say, that this was enough."

"Once, there was drought in that village. No one offered him food. Under the circumstances, the man and his family went without food for a whole week and were suffering from starvation. The husband and wife subdued their hunger by drinking water from time to time. But even their two young sons bore this difficulty without the slightest of squirm. This was truly surprising."

"After a week, he wandered around everywhere. Even then he stuck to his conditions without wavering. Understanding his plight, a generous woman gave him some flour."

"He brought it home and handed over to his wife. She made dough out of it and cooked four Rotis for the four of them. The children were eagerly waiting to eat after a long period of time."

"When all of them were seated for dining, a voice was heard, "Mother, I am feeling hungry, please give me something to eat."

"A figure of an old man appeared at the door. The body was skinny to the bones, the face had parched beyond recognition, which was covered with grey beard and moustache; the stomach had caved in for want of food for several days; the body was barely a skeleton."

"This was a family which lived on alms and did not consider the words, "Athiti Devo bhava" as merely a statement in the scriptures. So, the head of that family, without even second thoughts about it, gave away the roti that was his share to that old man."

"Eating by oneself, when there was a hungry guest at the door is against the scriptures, is it not? He did, what he did because of that."

"The old man sat at the door and after eating the roti, looked at them and said in a pleading voice, "Will I get one more Roti? I am unable to bear the pangs of hunger."

"The head of the family immediately looked at his wife. Without the slightest word, she handed over her share of one Roti to the guest."

"In this manner, the two of them, who had got something to eat after several days of starvation, gave away their food to a beggar. The story does not end here." The mongoose continued with the story.

"Mother, it has been many days since I ate any food. The Rotis that you gave me was like a morsel in front of an elephant sized hunger. Please give me something more to eat."

"When the husband and wife stood perplexed, not knowing what to do, the elder son handed over his share of one roti to the man. After finishing that as well, when the eyes of the guest was still dazed with hunger, the younger son also gave his share of one roti."

"The guest's hunger was appeased. But the two children fainted due to hunger. The Mother got agitated."

"The head of that family looked at the guest and asked, "Was your hunger satisfied?"

"My stomach had gone hungry since several days. That was why I had eaten all the food without even leaving anything for you" said the guest.

"Swami, was your hunger satisfied?"

"If it is not satisfied, what will you do?" asked the guest in return.

"Going against my principles, I will once again go to beg. Whatever I get, I shall bring and give you to satisfy your hunger" said the head of that family.

"Hearing this reply the guest was pleased and said, "Your approach to a guest is indeed very unique, elevating. I am extremely satisfied. Saying this, he stroked the two children who had fallen fainted there."

"They immediately sat up as though touched with a renewed energy. The guest left."

"The next moment the appearance of that house changed. It became wealthy. Grains filled the containers and overflowed. The house was filled with money and gold. They understood that the guest who had come there was a God of Dharma. He had come to test their approach to guests. They had won the test. The result was this overflowing wealth and prosperity. The husband and wife were overjoyed."

"Immediately, I rolled on the flour that was spilt on the floor of the kitchen of that house. That flour got stuck to only one portion of my back. That portion alone turned into gold. My surprise knew no bounds. At the same time, it even struck my mind, that what came to the hand could not reach the mouth. I even regretted. Only half my body was shining in gold; if only the flour had stuck to the whole of my body, my whole body would be golden in color. I felt that I deserved only that much and so felt contentment and regret at one and the same time."

"At that time there was an aerial announcement. This poor family has done a great yagna. Yes. Sacrifice. They sacrificed their own food to a guest who had come to their doorstep looking for food which is a greater sacrifice than the sacrifice in a yagna. Go to a yagna which is being done on a grander scale than this and roll in the flour that is scattered around in the kitchen area. The rest of your body will also turn gold" was the announcement."

"After that, it had become my practice to go to every yagna that took place and roll around on the flour that is scattered around that place. So far I have not had any luck. Hearing that this yagna was being conducted by Dharmaputra, I came here. Here too I have had to only face disappointment."

Hearing this, Dharmaputra and the Pandavas bowed down their heads.

Having seen the greatness of Shri Hayagreeva, the glory of conducting the Ashvamedha yagna, the pride of the horse used in the yagna, now we shall look into the writings in the ancient scriptures of the rituals involved in the worship of Shri Hayagreeva. We shall also see the not so well known secrets about Hayagreeva as well.

5

The rituals in the worship of Hayagreeva from the ancient scriptures

Hayagreeva has been worshipped in our country since ancient times. His importance and glory can be found in the Hayagreeva Upanishad, important Puranas and in the worship of Shri Vedanta Desikar and other great personalities.

Bhagwan Shri Krishna says in the Bhagawad Gita that among Mountains the highest is the Himalayas, among Purohits I am Vasishta, I am Brahaspati among Vedic scholars, and I am Muruga among the army leaders. I am Brahma among those who spread morality, I am Ahimsa among vows, I am the King among devotees, I am Hanuman among the wise, and I am Sanatkumar among Brahmacharis etc.

He further goes on to say that among those worshipful to the Vishnu devotees are Vasudev, Shankarshana, Pradyumna, Aniruddha, Narayana, Hayagreeva, Varaha, Narasimha, Vamana, the nine incarnations all of whom it is me, Vasudeva alone.

From this it can be concluded that Hayagreeva also was one of the incarnations of Shri Narayana.

The science of astrology indicates as to who are those who should worship him. Every star has a presiding deity and a deity for worship.

For example, for those born under the star, Ashwini, worship of Shri Saraswati will bring all kinds of success. Those born under the star Bharani should worship Durga. Similarly those born under Tiruvonam should worship Shri Mahavishnu and more specifically, Hayagreeva which will be very beneficial in removing all difficulties. They will enjoy all happiness.

This incarnation with a horse face and a body of man is hailed in the Mahabharata as Hayamukha. This idol has been worshipped in our country since very ancient times. There is evidence of this in the Upanishads. There is also references to him in the Agama literature, main Puranas, Four thousand Divine Prabandham and others.

Hayagreeva in the Puranas

In the texts on Vaishnavi Dharma we get references about Hayagreeva. He manifested from the primordial state of Shri Mahavishnu as an ansh of Vasudeva. He has the knowledge and capabilities of Shankarshana. He should be worshipped in the form with the face of a horse and eight arms. He holds the conch, chakra, lotus, staff in four of his hands and in the other four hands, he has the four Vedas. One leg is placed over Sri Devi as well, as described in this scripture.

The Agni Puran mentions Hayagreeva to be holding the conch, chakra, book, staff in four of his hands, his left leg is placed on Seshanag and his right hand is placed on a Tortoise. The same thing has been described in the Matsya Puran and Brahmanda Puran. However in the Brahmanda Puran there is a slight difference in the weapons held by Hayagreeva. He is described as having four hands in which he is said to be holding the conch, chakra, a book and Japa mala. The Japa mala has replaced the staff.

In the Garuda Puran, he is described as having a brilliant white neck which shines like white conch, white jasmine flower, white like the Moonlight cool and pleasant. His four hands have a white conch, chakra, a mace, and a lotus. His neck is adorned with a garland of wild flowers. He has sharp cheeks, beautiful and shapely mouth, and is wearing yellow colored robes as he gives his darshan.

Hayagreeva as in the Agama literature

The Agamas describe him to have two hands like man and sometimes he is also depicted as having four hands and still other Agamas mention him to be eight armed, and even twelve armed. According to the number of hands, the kind and number of weapons and tools in them vary.

By and large, the he is equipped with tools that are generally attributed to Maha Vishnu but he also carries some other things like Traces, Japa mala which are additional. The reason for this is his being the authority over education and knowledge.

The Sesha Samhita has elevated him to be the Creator as well. Besides, his body is also decorated with various kinds of ornaments; he is also seen carrying five chakras.

This form as the bearer of five chakras (Pancha Chakradhari) is not mentioned elsewhere.

The main deity with a horse's face and human body is seated on a white lotus. His face is shining like a crore suns. In one hand he is showing the Jnyana Mudra while the other three hands hold the book, conch and chakra.

Padma Samhita depicts him as having the face of a horse, the body of a man, wearing white robes, having four hands of which one is showing the Mudra of blessing, while in the other three hands, one carries the symbol of knowledge in the form of a book, the second carries the symbol of meditation in the form of a Japa mala and the third hand carrying the symbol of victory in the form of a white conch.

Parashar Samhita describes his appearance and the equipments in his hands in a slightly different way. He is shown as having two hands. He is seen wearing various kinds of ornaments. Besides, he is seen seated along with his beloved goddesses, Sri Devi and Bhudevi. His two hands are holding the chakra and a lotus.

Hind Samhita describes him as having fifteen hands which are carrying only five things namely the conch, chakra, mace, lotus and a book. The hands on Gods are depicted as two, four, eight, twelve etc. i.e. normally in pairs. But here the number fifteen is odd number which appears to be amusing.

Sometimes, the Noose, the goad, blue lotus, conch, chakra, book, mace are considered to be singular in number.

He is also depicted with eight hands when he is addressed as Ashtabahu Hayagreeva. Here he carries the conch, chakra, mace, lotus, bow, arrow, sword, and the noose.

The Agamas have depicted him holding various weapons that highlight his strength and have also attributed him with varying number of hands.

6

Mantras and Yantras

Since ancient times, mantras, Tantras and Yantras have been used in the worship of Shri Hayagreeva. Padma Samhita describes about how the picture of Hayagreeva is to be drawn on a copper plate along with the requisite mantras to be etched on it for the purpose of performing the puja. The Mudras of Hayagreeva and the abundant benefits that one will get from each of them are also underlined in this book. Our ancestors knew that extraordinary powers of knowledge can be attained through the use of this mantra vidya.

These ancient scriptures reiterate the efficacy of pronouncing these mantras properly and writing them correctly and systematically on the copper plate and performing its puja for being an instrument for attaining the grace and blessings of Hayagreeva.

Beauty in form

The Tantra books namely Shraddha Tilaka Tantra, Meru Tantra, Lakshmi Tantra, and Yogini Tantra, give the Tantric methods of worship of Hayagreeva. They also mention Hayagreeva to be the God who showers knowledge. It was he who had retrieved the Vedas from Asuric powers.

Shraddha Tilaka Tantra book describes Hayagreeva as a God with the face of a horse, having a neck white like the snow, cool like the Moon in winter, and one who is brilliantly white. He is beautifully and tastefully decorated with ornaments of white pearls, and conch shells. He is seen with four hands, two of which is placed on his thighs while the other two are holding the conch and the chakra.

This is the description that is comparable to the statues of Hayagreeva that is found in temples today.

Meru Tantra gives a description of some additional features of Hayagreeva. The mantras for his worship, diagrams of his Yantras, the rituals involved in their worship, the daily prayers also can be found in this book. The descriptions of his form depicts him to be of a calm countenance, handsome in appearance, strong armed and able bodied. The color of his body is like that of camphor. He holds the lotus and a book, in his hands. The Moola Mantra, one hundred and eight names, Hayagreeva Gayatri mantra are also found in this book.

The book by the title Yoga Tantra describes the mystical qualities of Hayagreeva and the steps to be followed for attaining those Siddhis. In the ninth chapter of this book the incarnation of Vishnu Hayagreeva and the rituals in his worship has been described. This Vishnu Hayagreeva is the same as Hayagreeva Madhava worshipped in the contemporary times. A famous temple dedicated to him is found in Hajo village in the state of Assam near the Manigutto Mountain. The glory of Hayagreeva is described here in the form of a dialogue between Shiva and Parvati. In the Shakti Upasana there is the left hand side worship of the Goddess which has also been mentioned in connection with the worship of Hayagreeva.

Direction of Hayagreeva

God Hayagreeva who showers knowledge on his devotees is well known for his strength, agility and a foundation of support. Some Agamas describe him as the Protector of forces. He is depicted in some places like the security force on the flag of the temple gopuram. In some temples he can also be seen amongst the family of gods in the outer corridors of the temple.

As per the Agama scriptures, every deity is assigned a position facing a particular direction. In that sense Hayagreeva is invoked facing the northern direction and his puja is to be performed as per the Vishwaksena Samhita.

In accordance to the Northern direction being allotted to Hayagreeva as per the Puja Vidhi, he is given the place in the north in the aerial gods on the Gopuram of the temple. Just as Hayagreeva is placed in the northern direction, Shridhar is placed in the Eastern direction.

Narada Samhita says that the idol of Hayagreeva should be installed in the second site of the Gopuram.

But the Vishwamitra Samhita states that Door keeper gods like him should be placed in the first site of the Gopuram. Thus along with Varaha, Narasimha, Shridhar, Hayagreeva should be placed facing the four directions. In some temples there is a place for Garuda too in some temples.

Generally, the aerial gods are considered as security guards for the directions as known to us. Kapinjala Samhita has accepted this to be so and places Hayagreeva as the Protector for the northern direction.

Sanatkumar Samhita emphatically mentions Hayagreeva as the Protector of the Northern direction.

Moreover, in the Vaishnavi Sapta Matru temples, we can see him among the line of Door keepers. The names of the Seven Matrus appear different in different Agamas. Generally they are known as Brahmi, Vaishnavi, Maheshwari, Koumari, Varahi, Mahendri, and Chamundi.

Narada Samhita mentions their names as Vaguleshwari, Kriya, Keerti, Lakshmi, Srushti, Vidya and Kanti as the seven Matrus. They grant their blessings standing facing the southern direction.

Further, it is also mentioned in the book that Sridhara and Hayagreeva as the two Door-keepers to the temple of the Seven Matrus are found as battle warrior Gods and are found either in the corridors of the temple or on the second site of the Gopuram.

In the Tantric tradition, every male God has a female goddess as his consort. Just as Shaakta has Shakti, Hayagreeva has Vaguleshwari as his female consort.

As the Family deities, Surya, and Chandra come in the second round. In other words they should be present close by as mentioned in one of the Agama scriptures.

The Supreme Being, Shri Narayana, among the Vaishnavas has incarnated in five states. They are Param(Supreme), Vibhavam (the celebrated), Vyuham (strategic), Archavatar (Ruling incarnation) and Antaryami (Present within).

Among these as Vyuham or strategic, the incarnations taken are as Vasudeva, Shankarshan, Pradyumna, and Aniruddha.

A book titled Lakshmi Tantra mentions the above four incarnations to have been manifested from Mahalakshmi herself.

The Puranas speak of the incarnation of Hayagreeva with the face of a horse as the incarnation of Vishnu himself. Some Pancha Ratra Agamas (practitioners of the Tantric rituals for five nights) speak of Hayagreeva as an incarnation of Shankarshana.

Here, Shankarshana was credited with knowledge and strength, Aniruddha for strength, and as an Authority over sharpness of intellect. Therefore, worship of Hayagreeva brings knowledge, and physical strength can be definitely deduced from this.

7

Hayagreeva Loka

The Hindu religion often speaks of seven Lokas or worlds. Among the Lokas seven of them are supposed to be above and seven below thus totaling to fourteen Lokas in all according to the Vedas and Puranas. Bhu, Bhuvar, Suvar, are some of the Lokas so also, there is the Dhruva Loka. This was created for Maharishi Dhruva. Similarly there is also a world in the name of Hayagreeva and is called the Hayagreeva Loka. It is believed to be an extension of the Goloka.

The Goloka is considered to be the dwelling place of Shri Krishna according to the Bhagavatam.

Goloka is said to be the place where Krishna, Radha and the other Gopis live joyfully as mentioned in the Puranas. This Loka is located in the upper part of Vaikuntha Loka which is the abode of the Supreme Paramatman. Wherever cows do not have a healthy habitat, in all those places, Shri Krishna manifested for blessing them as per the Bhagavatam. In that sense, Goloka was created by Shri Krishna out of his own desire and there can be no surprise in the fact that he dwells there willingly.

When the Devas and Asuras churned the Milk Ocean for getting the Nectar of immortality, a cow by the name of Kamadhenu also manifested. Along with her, five other divine cows named

Nanda, Bhadra, Surabhu, Sushila, and Kamani also appeared. These five cows also live in the Goloka. Shri Krishna and Radha are sustaining this world as the King and queen.

Those who construct a Rasa Mandapam install the idol of Shri Krishna and pray to him and sing his Bhajans is said to attain the Goloka after their time on the Earth as stated in the Brahmavaivarta Puran.

Uniqueness of Hayagreeva Loka

Hayagreeva Loka is a hundred yojanas in length and a hundred yojanas in breadth. This Loka is decorated with beautiful pearls all along its compound walls. There are four Gopurams made of gold. There are ten similar Lokas that encircle the Hayagreeva Loka from above, below and around. Hayagreeva Loka is located at its center and is ruling all of them from there. It is because of this Universe that more than a hundred red colored Universes exist simultaneously there.

In the center of Hayagreeva Loka there is a brilliantly shining mountain equivalent to a crore Suns. When one looks or thinks of this mountain, there is a joy that rises in the heart and there is a sense of peace. This mountain is called Lokaloka. A river by the name of Prasaravani originates in this mountain and gushes forth from there. There are several gigantic banyan trees on this mountain whose roots are hanging to the ground and from which more trees have grown. These banyan trees are so enormous that beneath the shade of each one several lakhs of horses, elephants and chariots can be stationed.

The circular path around the Lokaloka Mountain is called Tungakanti. It is very novel, beautiful and is the favorite among Munis and Rishis.

There are four huge Gopurams on top of the mountain. The names of the Gopurams are Niyam, Nivaya, Kalaya and Paralaya. The entrances to the four Gopurams are called Chandana, Pradhana, Sudana, and Dhana.

They are guarded day and night by four Door keepers. The South is guarded by Trinetra, the West is guarded by Kishana and Rohana, and the North is guarded by Pramoha and the East by

Vishwaha. They guard their respective directions like the eyelids guarding the eyes.

At a distance of 100 yojanas from the Southern Gopuram is the Soma Loka. This Loka extends up to a 100 yojanas. All the Lokas that we saw earlier including the Soma Loka, worship Shri Hayagreeva as the God of Protection.

In this manner, it is evident as to how important Shri Hayagreeva was as a deity of worship both as the Main deity and as the Family deity during the ancient times.

Hayam means horse. Now we shall look into his actual incarnation as a horse faced man itself.

8

Yagna Vishnu

Brahma is in charge of creation. A night in the life of Brahma is the period of Pralaya or annihilation of the world. When he wakes up again he begins his work of creation of this Universe. Once while he was asleep, the Vedas emerged from his mouth and fell outside.

These were gathered by an Asura named Hayagreeva and covering them up with his yogic powers took them to his Patala Loka and hid himself there. Hayagreeva had a human body and a horse face.

When Brahma woke up from sleep and he wished to begin his work of creation he could not find the Vedas that were necessary for assisting him in the task of creation. He was perturbed.

Immediately Brahma went to Shri Narayana and prayed before him. At that time, Madhava who had incarnated as a fish and was sustaining the world, assumed the form of Hayagreeva and manifested for the assistance of Brahma. He had assumed the same form of a horse faced man in this incarnation in order to defeat the horse faced Asura in battle. He dived into the waters and picking him out from his place of hiding, killed him. He retrieved the Vedas and restored them to Brahma. It was after that, that the work of creation began and the credit for that has been attributed to the incarnation of Hayagreeva by the Puranas.

Why did Mahavishnu select the face of a horse for this incarnation? Let us familiarize ourselves with some of the juicy reasons for this.

How did the horse face come about?

The incarnation of Mahavishnu as Hayagreeva has been described differently in different Agama scriptures, and Samhitas. What we saw earlier was one of them. In another version that has come up, Mahavishnu himself did not assume the form with the face of a horse for killing the Asura, but circumstances made that face come to him.

The story that we are going to look into presently is not from any Agama or Samhita. These have been gathered from bits and pieces found here and there and when put together we get the following sequence of events. Let us look into that as well.

Yagna Vishnu

Once in the distant past all the Gods desired to perform a very big yagna together. Since the fruits of the yagna was glory, fame powers and prosperity that was beyond imagination, all gods expressed their consent. The Gods decided to share the benefits that were to come from the yagna equally amongst themselves. On this condition and agreement the yagna began.

When this yagna took place at Kurukshetra, Mahavishnu, i.e. Yagna Vishnu alone did not desire that the fruits of the yagna should go to the others. Therefore during the yagna when the pot of sweet kheer emerged from the Agni Kund, he took it away from the Gods and deities present there, forcefully.

When the Gods and deities obstructed him, Mahavishnu drove them away with his bow and arrow. Indra, Vayu, Agni, and Varuna unable to oppose Mahavishnu, backed out. As a result of not only having transgressed the agreement arrived at before the yagna, but also having caused obstructions, the gods and deities got very angry with Mahavishnu and yearned to punish him.

They decided to punish him with the same arrow with which he had driven them away. When Mahavishnu stood vehemently ready to fight with the arrow mounted on the string, as per the directions of Indra, Vayu and Varuna converted themselves into termites and bit the string of the bow.

The string of the bow which was very stiff having cut off, the bow straightened. Since it had straightened very swiftly, it cut off the head of the person that was holding it, Mahavishnu. None of the Gods, including Indra and others expected this to happen even to the slightest extent. Their intention was only to teach Mahavishnu a strong lesson by breaking his bow. But the situation had turned upside down in an instant. They had never anticipated that his head would be cut off. All of them got frightened. In their panic, they looked at the Devaguru Bruhaspati for guidance to restore Mahavishnu back to life.

He called the Ashwini Kumars and instructed them to place the beheaded face of Mahavishnu back on his body. They agreed to do so on the condition that they should be given a jar of Soma juice in return. The reason for this request was that they were prohibited from having Soma juice.

Not having any other option, the Devaguru agreed. Immediately the Ashwini Kumars brought the head of a horse and attached it on the body of Mahavishnu. This was how Mahavishnu got a horse's face is the statements in some portion of the Vedas.

Charging evidence and the Madhuviddhai

The intention of narrating this story here is to lay the foundation for a deep subject which we are going to look into presently. The Ashwini Kumars were experts in surgery. Information about their extraordinary expertise in the science of transplanting organs into the human body and making them function smoothly may perhaps be astounding to many of us.

Let us look into how the incidence of surgery is closely interwoven with the knowledge of alcohol.

When the head of Yagna Vishnu was cut off, an alcoholic juice started flowing out of his body. Indra, who had arrived there first, seeing the alcoholic juice flowing from Yagna Vishnu's body, picked up some of the juice and applied it on his hands. He then applied it on his legs. As he went on doing this, his whole body began to look beautiful and shining. He attained the luminosity of Mahavishnu.

This act of Indra is termed as Madhuviddhai or science of alcohol. Anyone who possesses this skill can have the appearance of Mahavishnu very easily can be seen from the surgery incident.

There is another story related to this which appears in the Bruhadaranya Upanishad.

The head that has been separated due to having been cut off, or a head that is severed due to offering in a sacrifice can be once again joined with the body through the skilled use of the alcohol juice is something which Indra came to know of. He had learnt this skill from Tatyaga Muni himself. This Muni too had a horse's head. He had also threatened this Muni not to impart this knowledge to anyone else and had thus kept him under control. This has been mentioned in the Bruhadaranyaka Upanishad.

Even though Indra had threatened him in this manner, Ashwini Kumars had very cleverly received instructions of the skills of this knowledge of alcohol juice from Tatyaga Muni himself. That was why their services became presently useful for the gods.

Information about this Muni can be found in several places in the Atharvana Veda. This Muni who himself had a horse's head had taught the Madhu Vidya to Indra. With this knowledge it was possible to put back the heads of animals that were offered as sacrifice in yagnas and thereby bring them back to life again. After learning this knowledge, Indra threatened the Muni from whom he had learnt this knowledge not to teach it to others. If he ever did so, he would become the target of his wrath. Without having any consideration for his being even his Guru, he would cut off his head with the Vajra weapon he had warned him.

Ashwini Kumars approached Tatyaga Muni pleading with him to impart the knowledge to them. He told them of Indra's warning.

As a solution to this eventuality they said that he could teach them this knowledge by cutting off the head of a horse and then reinstating it to the body thereby demonstrating the application of this knowledge. If Indra, on coming to know of this were to cut the head of the Muni, they would then put the head of this horse on his head through the use of the Madhu Vidya. Tatyaga Muni too accepted this and did as was told. Indra came to know of it and cut off his head.

Immediately the Ashwini Kumars cut a horse's head and joined it to his body by applying the Madhu Vidhya and restored him to life. This story, described in the Upanishad says that since the Ashwini Kumar had foreseen what would happen and as it happened accordingly, they could get this knowledge.

It was in this context that when the head of Yagna Vishnu was severed, Ashwini Kumars were called to fix the horse's head on his body.

Now the doubt arises as to whether they only had the knowledge of fixing a horse's head to the human body and making it alive. That was why, in the beginning itself when they learnt the mantras, they used it in fixing a horse's head on the head of the Tatyaga Muni himself explains the Upanishad. Here also, Yagna Vishnu was given a horse's head alone by the Ashwini Kumars. Those who are interested in further research in this matter should keep this fact in mind before exploring further in order to find fruitful evidence related to this.

9

Why did the horse's face come about?

Devi Bhagavat gives a different story as to the reason for this. Brahmadeva once performed a one thousand Mahayuga Ashwamedha yagna. Vishnu agreed to see that he is not disturbed by any Asuric forces during the yagna. Vishnu set himself up adjacent to the Yagnashala where the yagna was being performed and stood there on guard with his bow named Sarangam without batting an eyelid. Nothing untoward took place. The Asuras dared not to enter anywhere near the yagnashala and frightened they kept to their corner.

After the completion of the one thousand Mahayuga Yagna, Brahmadeva came towards Vishnu to express his gratitude. At the end of the yagna, when he wished to offer his respects to him as well, he found him absorbed in deep Yoga Nidra. After having remained awake and vigilant keeping guard for the Mahayuga yagna, seeing him asleep, Brahma and the other Devas woke him up.

He did not wake up so easily. So they decided to use some push tactics to wake up Vishnu from his sleep. But they did not anticipate that such an act could turn adversely upon them.

Hoisting the bow, Vishnu was fast asleep leaning on it. However much they tried they could not disturb him from his sleep. So, they thought if they pulled aside the bow on which he was resting his hand, his hands would slip away and that would wake him up.

Yes. That was a good idea. How is that to be done asked Indra.

Brahma suggested, "I shall create termites. All they need to do is bite the strings on the bow and cut it off."

The Devas accepted the suggestion and encouraging him asked him to proceed accordingly.

Brahma created the termites and ordered the other Gods to go and get the strings of the bow cut down and wake Vishnu up from his sleep.

Immediately the Termites spoke, "Prabhu! If we wake Paramatman from his sleep, won't we be at the receiving end of his curse?"

According to the Shastras, it is wrong to wake someone up when he is fast asleep. Separating the husband and wife, or untying the sari of the mother, are all sinful acts and are subject to punishment. The same punishment is applicable for waking up someone during sleep. If we get more specific, the sin is equivalent to that of killing a person chanting the Vedas.

It was with these consequences in mind, that the termites had pleaded in that manner.

Brahma replied, "Yes, that is true. If, for our sake, you are agreeable to do the sin, then henceforth you too shall get a portion of the offerings to any yagna."

The Termites were happy. They cut the knot of the string on the bow. With the cutting of the string, the other end of the bow collapsed with a thud. In the force and the speed with which it came down, it cut off the head of Mahavishnu which fell into the yagna kund.

This incident that happened in just a fraction of a second, almost before the flash of an eyelid, left Brahma and the Gods present there as though thunder struck. They were stunned. They burst out, "What a tragedy this is! We had performed the Yagna for so many years and the very protector from difficulties, the guardian for the orphaned, the one who had shielded the yagna from any kind of obstacles all these years, we sacrificed that very person!"

All of them went and fell at the feet of Shri Lalita Parameshwari. They begged her to wipe away their sin.

She manifested before them in the form of Mahamaya.

She said, "O Gods! Do not distress! Cut off the head of the horse that was to be offered as the sacrificial cow in the yagna and place it on the body of Mahavishnu. Through that form he shall incarnate as Hayagreeva."

The Gods did as they were told and Shri Hayagreeva manifested.

The Goddess, looking at Hayagreeva, said, "An Asura with a horse's head, after doing penance to Lord Shiva for several thousand years has attained a boon from him that he shall be killed only by one who had the head of a horse like me. You have incarnated solely to kill him alone. That is the purpose for the happening of this incident."

She also added that Shri Mahalakshmi too had cursed him that he should have a horse's head and that is another reason for this happening, saying which she disappeared. The Gods profusely thanked her for having restored the head of Mahavishnu and brought his life back.

Mahalakshmi's curse

Puranas have the practice of quoting some curse or the other for questions whose answers are unknown. There is definitely a cause for every action. Sometimes we are not clear as to the purpose for the same. The cutting of Vishnu's head is also one such situation.

After the conclusion of several thousand years of a yagna performed by Brahmadeva during which period Mahavishnu was on guard ever vigilant so as to not allow any obstacles to come in the way of its performance until successful conclusion, there should actually have been benevolent results after the yagna, is it not? But that did not happen. Sometimes it happens like that. Those who do good not only go unrewarded, on the other hand they become victims of tragedy as well.

What is the reason for such happenings?

As far as human beings are concerned it could be explained by saying that it was due to some previous lifetime's bad karma, as explained by Astrological science.

What is the reason for Gods to also having to face such sorrows?

Nothing can happen without a reason. For a thing to happen there might have been some cause. So, Puranas use curse as the means of explaining the cause for such incidents in order to have a sense of satisfactory acceptance.

When a man is required to face some sorrow for no reason at all or he suffers a loss for no fault of his, he is disappointed, depressed and feels hopeless. In such situations, it is such incidents quoted in the Puranas that offer him some solace.

For example, when some women face sorrow in their lives, they get greatly dejected. "Why does this happen to me alone?" Brooding on this again and again they become subjects for depression.

It is during these times that historical stories become useful. Is there any sorrow that Sita did not face in the Ramayana? Was she an ordinary woman like any of us? She was Maharaja Janaka's daughter. In other words, after being the daughter of a Chakravarti, she had married to the son of another Chakravarti, Raja Dasharat, where she had begun to live.

There also, the man who married her was no ordinary youngster. He was Shri Ramachandra Chakravarti. Therefore, she had the backing of three Chakravartis and such an adorable woman had to face a livelihood like that of a wood cutter's wife? Having to go to the forest, she lived in a hut. How unfortunate her destiny had turned out to be. Doesn't it give a shiver merely thinking of it?

Can such a thing happen in the modern times to anyone? If it happens, will any woman bear it and sing the praise of such a husband and walk behind?

Sita had faced every difficulty with a pre-determined resolve. Have we faced with such kind of difficulties? We didn't. Then why should we get so dejected? We shall face it when it comes- that should be the attitude, is it not?

Similarly, in this situation, where Mahavishnu's head had been cut off, the curse pronounced by Sri Mahalakshmi at some point of time in the past became the cause as the story goes.

Once, when Mahavishnu and Goddess Lakshmi were seated alone, looking at her face, he happened to laugh loudly.

She asked, "Why are you making fun of me?"

"Nothing in particular, I just thought of something funny, and laughed." Vishnu replied.

Lakshmi asked angrily, "Does my face look funny?"

He did not reply but remained silent. That made her more furious.

Stating that he had been thinking of some other woman and that was why he was making fun of her, she started arguing with him.

However much he tried to convince her she would not listen. In the height of anger, she pronounced a curse, "Forgetting yourself, you looked at me and laughed. May your handsome face be cut off from your body and fall off."

What started off playfully, turned out to be ugly later in this manner. This is as unfortunate as the incident where the people who went to the exhibition of fireworks in celebration becomes victims of a fire disaster.

She had imagined in her mind that her husband was making fun of her having some other woman in his heart. Instead of leading a life with another woman as her competitive counterpart, it is better to live as a widow was the thought that was the reason behind this curse.

What is surprising here is that Lakshmi was angry at the thought that some other beautiful woman had come to steal her husband Vishnu away from her. In fact what happened was that a Devi with Tamasic tendencies had come looking for her. That is why she pronounced a curse that her husband's head would be cut off without even thinking what kind of humiliation, misfortune and sorrows of widowhood would befall on her as a result of that.

In spite of the fact that Mahalakshmi's curse was pronounced without prior thought or consideration, and without any enmity before hand, the curse ultimately proved beneficial in the end. But for the curse Hayagreeva's incarnation would not have taken place and as a consequence the Asura would not have been killed.

Apart from that, in the later years we would also not have got the benevolence of great persons like Shri Vedanta Desikar, Shri Vadiraja who had attained the blessings and grace of Hayagreeva. Therefore, if we consider these facts, even though things may happen which we do not like, and even if at that time we considered it bad, there will always be some good in that. We should bear our sorrows by thinking positive even in a negative thing. This is the lesson that we can learn from this incident.

The Asura's penance

The Asura Hayagreeva sat looking Goddess Sri Lalitambika incessantly for a thousand years with a single pointed devotion. Seeing this the goddess, pleased with his penance, manifested before him and said to him, "Ask for a boon that you desire."

He said, "Mother, I ask for the boon, that I be immortal. I should not die at the hands of any God, or any ghostly powers."

She replied, "That is not possible. Anything that is born in this world out of the five primordial elements is subject to death. Nobody can change this law. Ask for something else."

The Asura said, "If that is the case, then only a strange human being with a face of a horse should be able to kill me."

The Goddess blessed him with the boon saying, "So be it" and disappeared.

It is said that if a crab gets fat it cannot be contained within its shell. Similarly when the Asura got the boon his ego got inflated. "Who is there to confront me? Nobody can even get anywhere near me." Saying this he started creating trouble for the Devas and the Rishis.

Neither the Gods nor Indra could face him. He ridiculed them. The reason for his confidence was that only a man with a horse's face could kill him and he knew that such a person did not exist. Even their anger and valor became useless in front of him.

They got together and schemed a plan and accordingly the Goddess enacted it. It was because of this that Mahavishnu's head was cut off by the bow. Immediately the Devas approached Vishwakarma and prayed to him to affix a horse's head on the body of Vishnu.

He too, without wasting any time, found a horse, cut off its head and attached it to the body of Vishnu at the neck. It was in this manner that due to the grace of Goddess Mahamaya that the incarnation of Hayagreeva got manifested.

During the final stages of Kalpa period, the Universe was immersed in a deluge. Mahavishnu lay asleep in yoga Nidra on the leaf of a banyan tree floating on the waters. At that time from the dirt of his ears were born two Asuras, named Madhu and Kaitabh. These two Asuras considering themselves above Brahma himself, fought with him and grabbed the Vedas away from him.

Brahmadeva, not knowing how to proceed with the task of creation without the Vedas, approached Sri Devi Parashakti and expressed his difficulty to her. Ambika immediately disturbed Mahavishnu from his yoga Nidra. Mahavishnu then attacked the two Asuras and holding both of them on his thighs killed both with his chakra. Thus the death of the two Asuras has been attributed to the Goddess as per the Devi Bhagavat.

According to the Devi's wishes, Mahavishnu with the face of Hayagreeva saved the Devas by killing the Asura. In this way the Mahalakshmi's curse on him also was absolved. It is believed that those who read or listen to the reading of this portion of the Devi Bhagavat will be absolved of their sins. The obstacles faced by them will go away and prosperity will be restored. This is stated in the benefits of the reading in the Bhagavat.

Even today, the importance of the horse has not diminished from those ancient times. There are several explanations as to why Paramatman had to incarnate with a horse's head. We saw several clarifications from the Itihasas and Puranas. Even in practice the horse has been increasingly put to good use. Pulling the carts, travelling, drawing the chariots, for ploughing the fields, and even on the war front on the battlefields, horses have been used for years and years.

Even in the field of research and medicine horses are being used to a very large extent. Let us briefly look into that.

10

The stunning horse power

If one picks up any electric motor one can see the letters HP written on it. HP means horse power as we all know.

When we try to gauge strength of some animal, we look at the Lion, Tiger, and Elephant etc. who seem to have a lot of strength. Then why should the horse's strength be taken for measurement of the unit of strength?

The other animals may have strength but they do not have the speed. It may run very fast for a few minutes but soon they become breathless and stop to breathe. But a horse is not like that. With the white foam in its mouth, it has the capacity to keep running for several hours at a stretch without stopping.

In the early days of mankind, human beings used the horse to escape from other animals as they had to run away very fast. Man was easily chased and overcome by the animals. So he sat on the horse, trained it and learnt to ride over it. The speed that he was unable to muster up from his own body, he got by making use of the horse.

In this manner, man started adjusting his speed according to the needs of the changing times. Later he invented the wheel. He created the chariot with that. In order to pull those chariots at a great speed he attached the horse to it. Then he realized that four horses could pull a carriage faster than one horse. The chariot moved faster and this helped in attacking the enemies more speedily. The four-horsed chariot was calculated as having the power of four horses.

So, one unit of strength was related to the power of the horse to pull an object and thereby the method of using horse power as a method of calculation came into existence. With modernization the use of the words "horse power" increased in reference to strength. The strength of any invention made was gauged with reference to the strength of the horse power as the yardstick. Formerly these words were used only in the context of motor vehicles. But later it began to be used even in measuring the strength of electric motors.

When we say 400 HP it means it has the strength equivalent to the strength of the power of four hundred horses to pull some object. In the recent times, the use of horses has reduced but the measurement of its strength as horse power or HP has become permanent. From this you would have gauged the incredible strength and speed of a horse. Perhaps that was the reason why the Paramatman had assumed the face of the horse for his incarnation.

Prana Vayu is compared to a horse

In order to describe the process of the movement of Prana vayu, Shri Tirumoolanatha makes use of the example of a horse in one of his songs. It goes like this:

Aivarkku naayagan Avvoor Tulamaikal
Uyya Konderum Kudirai Matrondru
Meyyarkku Patru Kodukkum kodaadupoy
Poyyarai Tulli Vizhuthidum Taane.

The husband of five sense organs in the body is the Mind. There is a horse to ride over it. In order to take it to the desired destination and to carry it comfortably, this illusory horse is useful. To those who are truly deserving this horse can be ridden very easily. But for the untruthful, this horse can jump up and throw them down. So says Tirumoolar.

This song speaks of the use of Pranayama when done properly and the problems that can arise if not done at all. Here the word Oor indicated our body and the horse is symbolic of the practice of Pranayama.

Those who approach the Lord and the Guru with love at their center and staying near them learn the process of Pranayama with devotion and practice it diligently will become centered. Such people will be blessed with boundless horse power of Prana Vayu in the form of protection of the Guru and his blessings. However in the absence of the protection from the Guru and devotion to the Lord, if one thinks of controlling this horse, it will be like the water pumped into the fields, he says. This song indicates the enormity of skill and practice that is necessary to bring the speed and strength of a horse under control.

Nalan and horses of mind speed

Nalan was the King of the Nitatha Kingdom. His wife's name was Damayanti. Since he was caught by Kali Purusha, he lost his Kingdom, he lost his wife and children and without telling Rutuparna as to he was, he started living anonymously by the name of Vahuka, a puller of chariots which he has been carrying on for some time.

Damayanti, his wife, decided to conduct a Swayamvar to locate her husband.

When Rutuparna went to participate in the Swayamvar, Nalan pulled the chariot. Rutuparna ordered him to pull the chariot faster.

Nalan had the knowledge of the science of horses. He would say mantras for flying like the wind in the ears of the horses. In an instant the horses would fly in the air.

Due to the speed of the wind, the upper garment on the body of Rutuparna flew and fell to the ground.

Rutuparna said, "Vahuka, pick up the upper garment."

Before Nalan could pick up the garment, the chariot had covered a huge distance. Seeing this extraordinary skill of Vahuka in riding the chariot, Rutuparna asked him to teach that skill to him as well.

Nalan hesitated. Seeing this Rutuparna said, "Vahuka if you teach me the Ashwa Shastra, I shall teach you the science of Trees." He placed his request several times upon which Nalan imparted him the knowledge of the mantras that would make the horses gallop very fast and in return he learnt from Rutuparna the science of Trees. Learning this science, he could look at a tree and say how many branches, leaves, flowers and fruits the tree had. The biography of Nalan speaks of this splendid knowledge of the science of Trees.

Kings and horses

These types of horses have had strong relationships with the lives of several Kings. Armies of horses have been popular with Kings since very ancient times. The Kings in our country had won over great conquerors like Alexander, Napoleon and others due to the strength of their army of horses.

Since the times of Sangha, the Kings of our land had four kinds of armies: Chariots, Elephants, Cavalry and military. Here cavalry indicated the army of horses. Riding horses has been a science in our country referred to Ashwa Shastra learnt and practiced from eons.

In some of the ancient civilizations horses have been depicted as having wings and there are paintings of flying horses. These flying horses can be seen on flags, coins, official stamps and monuments. The Puranas speak of the chariots of the Sun and the Moon as having been driven by horses. In the Chinese calendar of astrology, of the twelve year cycle, the animal symbol pertaining to the seventh month is the horse. Even now, in our games of chess, the horse is considered an important part of the army, is it not?

Horses in medicine

In medical practice, in the research for cure against breakdown due to poison, horses are playing an important role. In order to counter act the snake poison, at first the medicine is injected to horses in a small measure. Counter acting to these certain chemicals are first injected into the horse's body. After they are mixed up in the blood, this blood is taken out and then they segregate the counteractive chemicals. This is used as the cure for snake poison caused due to snake bites in man.

In the earliest times of creation, the stolen Vedas were retrieved by Hayagreeva's incarnation. Similarly, in order that the human species is not destroyed due to snake poison, the horse becomes the sacrificial animal which is truly astounding.

Besides this, when people who are depressed or mentally challenged, get into close contact with horses, their mental confusion gets cleared and they regain their lost confidence. Along with medical treatment they get cured completely according to medical practitioners. It is for this reason that prisoners are assigned with the task of tending to the horses in the stable. As a result of this they become mentally cured and begin to lead a healthier and morally good life as per some medical reports.

The benefits from horses to humanity do not end here. The products made from horse's milk, and flesh is eaten by the Mongolian people. The urine of a horse that has recently conceived is used as medicine. The horse's skin is used for making gloves, shoes etc. It's broth is also used to make some kind of animal gum.

It is these several ways that horses have proved to be very useful for the human race, that perhaps Mahavishnu too assumed the face of a horse to incarnate as Hayagreeva in order to glorify this species, which thought would not be misplaced.

Just as the horses protect the Kings who ride them to the battlefield against their enemies to their last breath, the God who incarnated with a horse's face protects those who surrender to him and worship him with devotion, removing all obstacles and showers them with all kinds of endless possibilities and successes.

The incidents where Lord Shri Hayagreeva has played an important role in the lives of several great personages are innumerable. Let us look into some of them and get to know them better.

11

Hayagreeva's blessings on Yagnavalkya Maharishi

Veda Vyas had high regards for his student Vaishampayan. When the bundles of Vedas had increased beyond control, they were sorted and classified properly by Veda Vyas and the task of sorting the Yajurveda was given to Vaishamapayan.

His great devotee and student who studied the lessons from him was Maharishi Yagnavalkya. Vaishampayan and Veda Vyas taught the Vedas very systematically to Yagnyavalkya. He too learnt them in depth and with curiosity.

One day, a discussion ensued between Yagnavalkya and Vaishampayan on some issue. When the argument rose to its heights, the Guru got very angry and asked him to leave the ashram.

"Yes, surely, I am going," said Yagnavalkya.

Gurudeva said to Yagnavalkya, "You should go the same way as you came in. Therefore you should vomit all the Yajurveda that was taught to you and then go."

"That too is fine", said Yagnavalkya, and with his yogic powers gathered all the knowledge of Yajurveda that he had learnt, vomited it out and left. All the students of the guru transformed themselves into Titri birds and picking up the bits and pieces of Yajurveda vomited there, swallowed them. Titri means axe. This later became the Taittreya Samhita.

The language Titri in later times came to be known as Tathai. Tathai means parrot. Parrots repeat word for word what is said. Therefore Vaishampayans' disciples had behaved like parrots and therefore they had consumed the Yajurveda that was vomited by Yagnavalkya.

Will anyone consume vomit? Even listening to it churns the stomach; concluding that the Puranik stories are all so disgusting, people make crooked faces. If one tries to understand the story word for word, one is bound to have distasteful feelings.

It is necessary to absorb the essence of this story: differences of opinion had developed between Yagnavalkya and his Guru. Therefore they get separated. What lessons were taught about Yajurveda should not be kept to yourself and be used for your upliftment alone but should be taught to the other students who are present here. Share it with them and go. He could have told him in that manner.

Yagnavalkya would have then without going beyond the orders of his guru, could have stayed there for some more time and taught finer nuances of the Vedic mantras to the other students. They too without mincing words, and instead of feeling who is this one to teach us, that he is a student like just any one of us, could have learnt the mantras without leaving a single line and could have benefitted from it. This story in fact seems to have included these unsaid feelings behind it. The whole subject has been explained in the form of a story in a very delicate and indicative manner, is the truth.

After coming out of there, Yagnavalkya stood before the Surya Deva, the illuminator of all and did intense Tapas. Pleased with his penance Surya, gave a clue (under cover) as to how to retrieve the Yajur Veda which was in the form of Hayagreeva. Thus in order to retrieve the lost knowledge of the Vedas, the grace of Shri Hayagreeva was useful.

Among the horses that pulled the chariot of Surya, Vaji and Dadikra were very skilled. They had a portion of the strength of Hayagreeva in them. In the Sandhya Vandana Mantra, there are words such as "Dadikra Vanno, Jishnorasvasya Vaji". Through this, it was possible to understand the glory of Hayagreeva.

Receiving the benevolent glance of Shri Hayagreeva, the ocean of knowledge of all the Shastras, Yagnavalkya Maharishi was able to write the Yagnavalkya Smriti, in later times and thereby gained great prominence. He thus created the new Shukla Yajurveda. The earlier Vedas were called Krishna Yajurveda.

12

Shri Hayagreeva and Shri Bharatiraja

This is an incident that occurred about a hundred years ago. Towards the evening the cows that had gone to graze in the forests were returning home with their desires fulfilled. A young lad who had taken them to graze was also coming along with them. There was a divine glow on his face. The touch of the golden rays of the setting Sun shone on his face and body as though like a golden idol. Looking at the young boy, the people of the town became spell bound.

Overseeing the cows, the boy was returning to his home when a Palanquin drew up near him. The person travelling in it was the head of a Mutt. His name was Svarna Varna Parashurama Tirth. He asked the bearers of the palanquin to halt for a while. He called out to the young lad who was lustrous with a divine glow. He asked him, "How far is the village of Appur from here?"

"Look at me, look at the herd of cattle, look at the Sun as well, you will understand the truth", he said with a little mischievous twinkle in the eye as though covering the truth in a subtle way.

What audacity for a lad of such a young age! He was the Chief of such a big Mutt. Instead of giving a straightforward to answer to such a great person with due respect, the boy had blabbered something else made the palanquin bearers furious.

Some of them even admonished him.

The chief of the Mutt stopped them. Understanding the subtle mind of the young lad, he contemplated on his words. This is a diamond, this valueless diamond's place is not in this village, he concluded.

A wise man alone can understand a wise person, is it not?

The impressive Divine countenance of the boy had already captured his attention and then his playful intellect made him to come to a firm and benevolent decision.

It was twilight, an innocent boy, he has been grazing the cows the whole day and returning, which means that the Appur village could not be very far away. This is what the boy was saying in a very mysterious way.

On reaching the village, the Madhva Matadhipati, enquired about the young boy and sent a man to look for him.

The young boy belonged to Appur village. His real name was Lakshmi Narayanan. His mother and father were great devotees. They understood that they belonged to Mysore Chennapattinam Taluka.

Understanding that Paramatman Shri Krishna had begun his Leelas, he sent men to bring the parents of the young boy with due respects.

He enquired about their well-being. They were a little disturbed that such a great personage as the Matadhipati had called for them, was speaking to them, was giving them respect and glorifying them. They were a little frightened too.

What happened was just what they had been afraid of. The Matadhipati looked at them and asked, "Is he your only son?"

"Yes" they replied.

"This son is a treasure that is not available to anybody. Such a wealth as him should not be confined to one family alone." He said.

Both of them with their hearts racing, looked at each other.

"So what, Swami?"

Softly came the father's reply.

"So, give him for the Shri Mutt. Not only me, the entire country be grateful to you. It is not me saying this. It is the Paramatman's Divine intention. I am only conveying it to you." Said the great one.

The parents were silent.

The Matadhipati re-iterated, "The whole world is going to celebrate him. Because of him, the arts, and Madhva traditions will spread far and wide like the Banyan tree and give cool shade to all. Therefore if you understand the Divine Providence, everyone will benefit from it."

Even great Matadhipati gets praised by the people. When such a person as the golden colored Parashurama Teertha was praising their son, even the parents could not say anything. If this is God's will, then can it be changed?

With tears of joy in their eyes, they offered their beloved son to the Shri Mutt.

On an auspicious day, the boy was anointed with the title Lakshmi Naryana Teertha and was initiated into the Sanyasa Ashram.

That boy of knowledge was taught all the Shastras by Parashurama Teertha. The young lad with an intellect like camphor quickly absorbed everything. Just like several small streams flow to join the ocean, all arts on their own flowed towards him and got absorbed in him. Was he not a Divine child?

Some time passed. To one who was to grow and spread like a huge banyan tree, the lessons that could be given by him alone was not enough was the conclusion arrived at by the great one. After learning all the Shastras and then further attain authority over them and later to attain glory, he sent him to the Gurukul of Shri Vibhutendra.

He too, when he had learnt all kinds of Shastras with all doubts clarified, from the Acharya's Mutt, and was returning, a miracle happened.

Sri Raghunatha of Shri Uttarati Mutt arrived at the Mutt. He saw Lakshmi Narayana and was astounded at the way he learnt the Vedas.

"Who is this lad, who had Divine blessings? He seems to have such a magnetic power in his eyes that they are able to hold the people in its vision. The shining luster of his body has such a divine beauty in it. It is such a pleasure to watch the way he is learning and the way he is expressing them after understanding them. What a divine bliss it is to watch him! Who is he?", Sri Raghunatha asked.

"He is a precious gift from the Divine to our Mutt, his name is Shri Lakshmi Narayana" began Shri Vibhutedra and gave him all the information about him.

"Even after gaining all this knowledge, he is so restrained. He is the proof of the saying, "Pride always bows down". The sharpness of his intellect and his cleverness astonishes me." After grandly praising him in this manner and calling Shri Laxmi Narayanan near him, he said, " I shall ask you some questions. Will you answer?"

"I shall answer" came the reply from Lakshmi Narayana.

After quoting some statements from the Nyaya Shastra, he asked him to explain the meaning of some words.

Immediately came the reply, "The essence of the whole book is that itself." Hearing this, Shri Vibhutendra stood with horripilations all over his body. Shri Raghunatha exclaimed, "Aha, Aha!" He was overjoyed. He called Lakshmi Narayana and blessed him.

He could not hide his astonishment. "Such wisdom at such a young age! You are the very copy of Vyasa Bhagwan himself in the form of a youth!" He praised him in this manner.

Hearing these words, Lakshmi Narayana bent his head with humility.

Looking at Shri Raghunatha, he said, "You are Shri Pada, I am only a student. I have now come to learn at the Shri Mutt. Am I deserving of so much praise?"

Immediately, Shri Raghunatha said, "We are only Shri Pada. But you are truly the King to all Shri Padas. This is the truth. It is not merely praise. From today, you shall be known by the name of Shri Padaraja." Lakshmi Narayana got the name of Shri Padaraja since then.

Such a one as he had so much knowledge and wisdom that he had to face trouble at times from his enemies. However great a personage may be, such dangers and troubles cannot be escaped from. Is that what is called karma?

In those turbulent times, how Shri Hayagreeva came and helped Shri Padaraja, we shall see presently.

Shri Hayagreeva's idol that came walking

Just as the fragrance of Jasmine flowers spreads all over the garden, so also the knowledge and humility of Shri Padaraja spread across several places. Just as the fragrance of jasmine flowers is carried by the passing breeze filling several places with the sweet fragrance, so also, Shri Padarja's glory was carried forth by his students, volunteers, and devotees all over the country.

After seeing something nice, forty people enjoy the sight, sill there will be some four people who feel jealous. Isn't that natural? If that is the case with ordinary people, then in the case of a personage as great as Shri Padaraja, seeing his popularity, how many Pundits, whistlers, smooth talkers would be burning with jealousy? It happened exactly like that.

His fame had spread up to Kashi. The Pundits there were not appreciative of him and more particularly the fame that he had got and the respect that people and the politicians showed towards him. They were jealous to the extent that they even said they did not want to hear the mention of his name itself and finish him off.

It is shocking is it not? If the fame reaches boiling point, then he could be invited for a debate and won over-this thought did not occur to them. They planned to somehow or the other kill him. Evil people think of destruction alone, is it not?

Shri Padaraja went to Kashi. The people and the King received him with great honour and respect.

The Pundits had invited him to a debate. He too had agreed.

What was the subject of the debate?

It is possible to know only if told is it not?

The Pundits said, "Shri Padaraja, you are very intelligent, we know. Therefore, if you get defeated in the debate, you should jump into the Ganges and drown yourself in front of everybody.

Is it so?

Yes. Are you frightened?

Not afraid, but in case you get defeated, then will all of you jump into the Ganges and drown yourselves.

"What kind of a foolish question is this? Till date we have never lost a debate", they said.

"Okay, if in case that happened, then the condition that you have imposed upon me would become applicable to you all as well, is it not?"

That is not possible. All of us will leave our homes and embrace abstinence, said the Pundits cleverly.

"If it is a debate, then shouldn't the condition for the proposition and opposition be the same? Okay you are behaving like hypocrites, I can understand that. In spite of that I am accepting your condition and still agreeing to participate in the debate" said Shri Padaraja with generosity.

"For heaven's sake! Accepting such a self-defeating condition, Shri Padaraja is definitely a fool" was the thought in the minds of some people who rejoiced at this.

Shri Padaraja then announced that the next day the debate would begin before the King in his State Council's hall where we shall commence our proposition and opposition.

No! No! How can we invite the King for such a trivial matter? He may have several other important engagements. We shall ourselves arrange this debate in a temple hall said the pundits.

Shri Padaraja accepted even that with a smile. When we have the protection of the Divine, there was no need to be afraid of any enemy, is it not? Having understood this very well, he agreed to the debate with joy.

Even though the Pundits wished that the King need not know about the debate, somehow the news had reached the ears of the King through someone. He was not agreeable to the Pundits behaving partially. Let us give them a free hand and see what happens. If Shri Padaraja becomes distressed in any manner, I shall interfere and impose the rules. Thinking in this manner the King remained silent. But he did not get a chance for that.

The debate took place as scheduled. The Pundits faced a humiliating defeat. Now they had no way out. "We were defeated"; they could not say, they were not willing to accept the consequences. The reason being, they knew that all news regarding the debate would go to the knowledge of the King.

If they acted against the law, they knew that they would not be able to escape from the legal punishment. Hence they bore the loss like a thief bitten by a scorpion. Yes, all of them accepted abstinence.

By merely wearing ochre robes, is it possible to abstain from worldly activities. All of them did wear ochre robes, but they had not reached the level of mental maturity necessary to practice abstinence. Their mind and hearts were still filled with anger, vengeance, which went on increasing day by day. They pledged to somehow kill Shri Padaraja and swore that they would not back out from that decision.

When they attacked straight forward from the front they had faced failure. Now the only way out was to attack stealthily. They decided to adopt Tantra and mantra to use against him.

Yes. Making use of the power of mantras, they got the mouth of Shri Padaraja locked up. Due to the power of mantras he was unable to speak. His tongue would not move.

Understanding what the sorrow that had happened to him, Shri Padaraja started chanting the mantra of Shri Hayagreeva and praised him. He could only say the mantra mentally. He could not open his mouth and pronounce it loudly.

Then a strange thing happened.

An idol of Shri Hayagreeva manifested there in the form of a statue and it moved here and there. Seeing this, the people and the King were overjoyed. The fake pundits were hit on the face.

The spell of the mantra of the pundits was broken. Seeing the return of Shri Padaraja's speech, the whole town was astonished. Seeing his glory, the idol bowed. The statue of Shri Hayagreeva came to life for the sake of Shri Padaraja and came walking, much to the surprise of all the people. They patted their cheeks and shed tears of joy.

With the darshan of Shri Hayagreeva even though the mouth lock was broken and his speech had been restored, Shri Padaraja was moved deeply.

"Swami had manifested for my sake and had himself come and given me his darshan. How merciful he is. Enough of moving around, now please assume a seat and remain permanently for blessing us. Saying this he started chanting stotras in praise of the Lord.

This idol is present even to this day in the Shri Padaraja Mutt in the puja place.

In a place called Mulupagal near Bangalore in the Narasimha Kshetra, on the banks of the river, in the year 1486 he attained the feet of the Paramatman. There is the Brindavan of Shri Padaraja and the Narasimha Teertha. All can visit and seek blessings.

Among the several blessed personages in our country, who have received the grace of Shri Hayagreeva in its totality, Shri Vadiraja was also one among them. It would be beneficial to look into his life story and glorify it.

13

You will beget a son

Born and brought up in the Udupi district of Karnataka, where a majority of the people came to worship Lord Shri Krishna, Shri Madhvacharya was engaged actively in spreading teachings of the Madhva principles among the people and directing their minds towards God for which he had established nine Mutts. One among them is the Sothe mutt. The Matadhipati was Shri Vageesha Teertha.

One day a couple came looking for him. They were Devarama Pattar and Gouribai.

Looking at them gave an impression that they were very well to do. But there was something that was troubling them. Something was eating their hearts away like the termites which was evident from one look at their face.

If this was evident for even ordinary eyes, to one who was spreading the Madhva tradition, to one who had dedicated his entire life for the Sanatana Dharma, would it not be clear to such a great personage as Shri Vageesha Teertha?

Still, as though he wanted to allow the couple to explain things themselves at their own pace, he welcomed them and blessed them graciously.

Gouribai's eyes flooded with tears as though water has been let out from a closed dam. "It is the Lord who is everything for me. Still I am not blessed with a child. Although several years have passed since our marriage, and even after having visited several temples, prayed in different ways, performed several penances, observed vows, none has been useful so far. This shortcoming is eating into us and costing us our peace" saying this she concluded.

The great personage, looked at them and said calmly, "Your desire will be fulfilled. Leave aside all worries. However…"

Their faces had lit up when he had said that their desire would be fulfilled. But hearing the word however, their hopes filled face fell as though from the heights of a mountain top to a valley beneath. With eagerness and a little anxiety they pleaded, "What is it Swami? Please tell us."

He said, "You should give that child to our Shri Mutt".

Even their eyes were expressing what their mouths wanted to say, "What kind of a test this is?" It was as though the eyes that were given the vision were immediately being removed. They said, "Swami, we came to you for help since we had no children. But without having the joy of raising the child, we are feeling very sad to give him away to the Mutt."

The great one closed his eyes and went into meditation for some moments. After some time, he opened his eyes and said, "Alright, if the child is born within the house, he is yours and if he is born outside, he belongs to the Mutt."

They felt relieved. If somehow they will be blessed with the treasure of a child, that was enough; it was possible to keep the wife safely at home and take care of her. Arriving at this conclusion, Devarama Pattar nodded his head in agreement. Shri Vageesha Teertha gave the joyous couple some specific mantras and instructions as to how to chant them along with some Akshata and blessing them he sent them away.

The sage's words came true. Gouribai became pregnant. Devarama Pattar took utmost care of the mother and child to be. He did not allow her to go out of the house for any reason whatsoever. She too willingly and happily agreed to it. If the child happens to be born outside the house, he had to be given away to the Mutt was the condition agreed upon. The couple were bent upon preventing that from happening with all their powers. Months passed by and the time for delivery was drawing close.

One day some unavoidable guests arrived. They cooked and fed them with delicious food. Gouribai happily served the food on plantain leaves. When they were eating the food, a cow happened to come inside the backyard where it started eating the plantain leaves. It gobbled up the vegetables that were spread around.

Gouribai immediately went to drive the cow away. As though turning back it turned away, but immediately returned to start grazing at the plants there.

Gouribai, picking up a stick and shouting at the cow started driving her away. She lifted the stick as though to hit. It started moving slowly to go outside. Fearing that it might come back again, she continued driving it away to a certain distance. Without realizing she went outside the house.

When she realized that, immediately she panicked, "Oh! What did I do? In a hurry to drive away the cow, I forgot my resolution. I have come out of the house." She hurriedly turned to go back to the house, when all of a sudden she developed an excruciating pain shooting through her lower abdomen and she held on to her stomach tightly.

She instantly sat down there screaming, "Amma!". She bit her teeth to bear the pain attempting to get back into the house. But god's wish was different. She could not even drag herself. Hearing her frightful scream, Devarama Pattar and the guests rushed outside.

They saw Gouribai under a tree writhing with delivery pains. In another instant she gave birth to a beautiful lustrous boy.

Having already known about the coming birth of the boy through Divine vision, Shri Vageesha Teertha, called for some officials of the Mutt and sent them to their house with a golden plate. They arrived at the place in time to see that the newly born child instead of being placed on the floor, was immediately placed on the golden plate bearing which they brought the child. This is the story according to the Karna tradition.

Since the child was born outside the house, as per the condition, they handed over the child to the Shri Mutt. Congratulating the couple, Shri Vageesha Teertha said, "You have given away your first child to the Shri Mutt. Another son will be born to you. You can fondle and enjoy bringing him up" he assured. He offered them holy water and Prasad and blessed them.

The couple returned home happy at having got two mangoes with one stone.

The child that was offered to the Shri Mutt was bathed with the milk offered as Abhisheka to the Deity of the Mutt. He was nurtured and fed with ample knowledge and given all the motherly care and attention by Shri Vageesha Teertha. That child which enjoyed the blessings of Shri Hayagreeva to the fullest extent and performed many miraculous deeds was none other than Shri Vadiraja Teertha. He sang many keertanais under the pen name of Hayavadana. He became the Peetathipathi spontaneously and spread the Madhva tradition.

During his life time he has demonstrated an extremely miraculous incident pertaining to Shri Hayagreeva. Let us get to know that auspicious story and become blessed.

14

The mysterious horse that appeared at night

Shri Vadiraja Teertha who was born in a place called Heevinigere in the Udupi district of the state of Karnataka, became the pontiff of the Turavaram Poondu Mutt at the young age of eight. He studied under Shri Vageesha Teertha. An obedient and intelligent student, he soon gained mastery over Kannada and Sanskrit languages.

He had tremendous skills, unparalleled knowledge of principles, and ability to write Stotra books which kept on increasing with time. The books written by him are innumerable. He had great devotion to Shri Krishna of Udipi. The rituals and traditions framed by Shri Vadiraja are being practiced at that temple even to this day.

When Shri Vadiraja was the pontiff of the Sothe Mutt, there was a very huge privately owned land adjacent to the Mutt. The owner of the land grew grams on that farm. The crop too had grown to a considerable height and was ready for cutting. The crop had shown a fuller growth than normal and the owner was thinking of getting the crop harvested in a couple of days and accordingly went around the farm and looked at the crop closely.

The next day when he went to the farm, he was shocked because one side of the crop was entirely crushed. He realized that some animal had encroached on the farm at night and had been rolling around on top of the crops and crushed them. He tied the fence tightly and returned home.

The next day he went before dawn to have a look at the farm. When he saw a similar scene of some animal having crushed another portion of the crop he was burning with anger. He decided that he shall keep a watch that night and catch hold of the animal that was wandering into the farmland and crushing the crops merrily. He had a good mind to tie it up and give a good beating. Accordingly, he came at night and lay on a pile of hay waiting for the animal that was stealthily coming into his farm.

Around midnight, a white shining horse was seen coming out of the Shri Mutt and coming royally into the farm grazing. Seeing the beauty of the horse, he got so absorbed in it, that forgetting the purpose of his hiding he even forgot to drive it away, instead he sat there enjoying the sight. After some time he became alert and chided himself for being so absorbed in relishing the beauty of the horse instead of driving it away. He picked up his stick. Immediately he changed his opinion.

This horse belonged to Shri Mutt. Why drive it away? A connection with a big place will be more beneficial. Thinking that he would speak to the officials of the Mutt the next morning, he returned home.

The next day morning the owner of the land came to the Shri Mutt and meeting the officials narrated all that had happened.

When Shri Vadiraja heard this, he looked at him lovingly and said, "It is possible that according to what you have narrated, a white horse may have come and grazed on your farm. But that horse does not belong to the Mutt."

"No, Swami. That horse came from within the Mutt and I saw them with my own two eyes."

"That is not possible."

"I am telling you the truth. What I saw is true."

"What I am saying is also the truth. The reason is that, I do not have any horse in the Mutt" said Shri Vadiraja.

When he heard this, the land owner was shocked.

"Swami, what I say is the truth. Anyway, I shall keep a watch tonight as well and tell you tomorrow" the landowner said frightfully and went back.

He stood on guard at night. A white horse came out from within the Shri Mutt and entering the field, started grazing on it. After allowing it to graze for some time, the landowner, started shouting to drive it away. In an instant, it picked up speed like the wind and ran towards Shri Mutt. It went inside and disappeared.

The landowner who had followed the horse driving it away, thought at first of entering the Shri Mutt and telling the Swami of the truth then and there. He then realized that this being an odd hour, waking up such a great person who must be in deep sleep and that too for such a petty reason, would be inappropriate and so returned home.

The next day he met Shri Varadaraja and complained.

Realizing that there was some justification in the complaint of the landowner, Shri Varadaraja said, "Do not worry. I believe what you say. In the same way, you also believe what I say. There are no horses reared in the Mutt. There is something mysterious going on here. This is known only to that Lord Hayagreeva."

The landowner humbly implored, "Swami, I was unable to bear the loss by destruction of the grams crop on the field and that is why I spoke with such emotion. Please forgive me."

"No one should be at a loss due to the Shri Mutt. Therefore I shall reimburse whatever loss you have incurred. Go back without any worry" said Shri Vadiraja.

"Thank God! What damage occurred was not entirely lost! What does it matter whose horse it is? Whatever I have lost, I shall get back." Rejoicing at his good fortune, the land owner returned to his house.

The next morning, he went round the farmland. He was in for a surprise.

He went running as fast as he could and meeting Shri Vadiraja, he said excitedly, "How can I tell you about this surprise! Wherever the crop of grams had been trampled upon and crushed, the whole place has a crop of golden grams on it. What kind of mystery is this!" he exclaimed.

Shri Vadiraja closed his eyes and went into meditation.

He then said, "This is not an ordinary horse. It is a Divine horse" and smiled.

"Yes Swami, there is no doubt about it. This is a Divine horse. When I drove it away, it went into the Shri Mutt and disappeared mysteriously. When I complained that I had met with a loss, it returned in the form of golden grams" said the landowner with great amazement.

"The shining white horse that had come on your farm and grazed on the crop of grams was verily Shri Hayagreeva himself" said Shri Vadiraja.

"Oh Swami! I did wrong Swami! Swami, I thought it was an ordinary white horse and drove it away. I thought of it as an animal that has come to destroy my crops. I should not go of such opportunity due to ignorance again. This night Shri Hayagreeva will come to graze on my farm. I shall definitely see him and get my desires fulfilled."

"That is exactly what you should not do! If you look at that Divine horse today, you will lose your eyesight!"warned Shri Vadiraja.

"It's alright Swami! My goal itself is to have His darshan!" He said with a definiteness of purpose.

That night the landowner kept vigil on his field. At midnight the white horse came out of the Shri Mutt in a grand manner and entering the field started grazing on the crops. Wanting to have a closer look, he went near the horse. The next instant he lost his eyesight.

He did not regret that. He relished on the fact that, God himself had come in the form of a horse and had been grazing on his farm and he had seen that, and with that Self-satisfaction he lay down there itself. The next morning his servants came and took him home.

When Shri Vadiraja came to know of it, Shri Vadiraja prayed to Shri Hayagreeva to restore the eyesight of the landowner. Listening to his prayers, the Lord blessed him accordingly.

When the landowner got back his eyesight, his joy knew no bounds.

"Swami, the land on which the Divine horse had come from the Shri Mutt and trampled upon now belongs to the Shri Mutt itself," saying this, the landowner gave away that land to the Shri Mutt.

Since, then, the grams grown on that farmland is cooked and mixed with grated coconut is offered as Naivedya to the Lord. This practice was begun by Shri Vadiraja. That naivedya is called Hayagreevapandi.

15

Hayagreeva in green color

Hayagreeva, in order to spread the glory of one of his most favorite devotees, came as a white horse and not only granted His darshan to the landowner, but also restored the lost eyesight. If this was a miracle, then what can be said about the arrangement he got done through Shri Vadiraja to have his food as Naivedya by himself assuming the form of a horse and consuming the grams. This is a greater miracle is it not?

Now let us look into another miracle that is far- fetched from what the Divine horse had done.

Ever since that day, Shri Vadiraja ensured to offer the Hayagreeva Pandi as Naivedya to Shri Hayagreeva. The idol he had with him had a hidden mystery to it. Let us get to know about that first.

A sculptor was once engaged in making an idol of Vinayaka in Panchaloham (alloy of five metals). He mixed the metals in the right proportion and poured it into the mould. When he took it out after cooling, he found that the statue was that of Shri Hayagreeva instead of Vinayaka.

Surprised at the outcome, he once again filled the mould. Once again the horse faced Hayagreeva emerged from it.

Heart-broken, the Sculptor, lay down, a bit concerned. That night he had a dream in which he heard a voice which said, "Do not worry, hand over this statue to Shri Vadiraja of Sothe Mutt."

He did as per the voice instruction. It is the same idol that Shri Vadiraja worshipped with daily puja, performed with utmost devotion and offering of Hayagreeva Pandi Naivedya. It is also called Hayagreeva Matti.

Every day, the Naivedyam prepared for the Lord would be taken by him in a plate carried with both hand over the head. It is unbelievable that, Shri Hayagreeva would manifest as a white horse and with his front two legs placed on the shoulders of the devotee eat that Naivedya. He would even leave behind a little portion of the Naivedya as Prasad for the devotee. That true Prasad was what Vadiraja too ate. The public who saw Shri Vadiraja take the plate with the Naivedya and bring it back with a little remainder in it daily, began to have a little doubt.

In this Kaliyuga is this true? Which God comes in reality and partakes of the Naivedya offered? They sneered.

Some jealous people said, "Nothing of the sort is really happening. He himself is eating the Naivedya and putting the blame on God."

"Does he have to do such things to show off that he is a great devotee? Isn't it shameful?" retorted some mischief mongers.

Just as the dogs barking at the Sun, Shri Vadiraja paid no heed to these comments made by the people.

This infuriated them further and some people who became extremely jealous decided to get rid of him.

One day they mixed the Naivedya that was being offered as Hayagreeva Pandi with poison.

They planned to kill Shri Vadiraja who taking the name of the Lord would eat the Prasad of the Naivedya offered as Hayagreeva pandi.

But will the Lord allow that to happen?

On that day too like every day, Shri Hayagreeva manifested as a horse and considering that to be a special day, consumed the entire Naivedya, leaving nothing behind.

"What is this? This seems to be quite unusual. Daily God would leave a little of the Naivedyam behind for me, but why did he do this today?" these questions kept disturbing Shri Vadiraja.

The next moment, the white horse fell unconscious. Due to the intensity of the poison that had spread to the whole body, it turned green in color. It was then that Shri Vadiraja realized that something untoward had taken place.

"He was distressed. Bhagawan himself had consumed the poison that was meant for me? Am I as important as that? I am merely a genetic being is it not?" he cried.

Immediately, Vadiraja cooked a dish with the vegetable named Kulla, a variety of brinjal and fed it to the horse. On eating that, the white horse regained consciousness and got up.

Even then, Shri Vadiraja cried, "Wasn't it because of me that you had to experience such difficulty?"

"Vadiraja do not regret! It was to demonstrate the glory of your devotion that I enacted this play," convinced Shri Hayagreeva. It was then that Shri Vadiraja sort of felt alive again. As an evidence of this incident, we can still see a ring of green around the neck in the idol of Shri Hayagreeva.

Every year in the month of Avani according to the Tamil calendar, on the day of the star Tiruvonam is Shri Hayagreeva Jayanti. If on this day this Naivedyam is prepared and offered during worship, one will be blessed with all knowledge and learning.

One can get a long life and be blessed with health, wealth and happiness. Every month, on the day of Star Tiruvonam, Hayagreeva pandi can be prepared and offered as Naivedyam. Those who do this will have all growth, prosperity and will lead a glorious life on Earth.

Shri Vadiraja lived for several years after that, worshipping the idols of Shri Krishna and Shri Hayagreeva. In the year 1600, he entered the Brindavan at the Sothe Mutt, and ever since, he is believed to be blessing his devotees even today.

Even in this Kaliyuga, that Hayagreeva would come as a horse, that he would eat the Naivedya, all these are all merely cooked up stories: there are even those who speak of these incidents in this manner as well. As evidence for such people, we give below the required information.

Shri Ram arrived

There are people who say, there was no Shri Ram at all. Yet, evidences of his visit to Tamil nadu are being found from time to time and this is one of those.

Vishwamitra Muni took Rama and Lakshmana to a forest named Tillaivan where he conducted a very big yagna. When someone is performing an auspicious function, there would be someone who would cause some trouble, is it not? A queen by the name of Tataka caused obstruction to the yagna and prevented from its taking place smoothly.

She threw flesh, blood, and such other impure substances and defiled the newly made Yagna Kund. She threatened the Munis and drove them away. Vishwamitra brought Rama and Lakshmana in a bid to control her.

When Vishwamitra asked Rama to kill her, He hesitated a bit; the reason was that she was a woman; how could he kill her? Is it not a sin to kill a woman?

Understanding the mind of Rama, Vishwamitra said, "Her body alone looks like that of a female. She is a stone hearted creature. She kills living beings without the slightest of mercy. Therefore, killing her will not bring any sin. End her life without any hesitation."

Rama killed her and saved the Munis thereby enabling them to complete their rituals. The sin of killing a woman being equivalent to killing of a Brahmin haunted Rama and Lakshmana. In order to make amends for this sin, they performed a yagna at a place called Vijayapati. About three hundred years ago this place was a big flourishing town. Presently this town is divided into two villages and can be seen as Vijayapati Melur and Vijayapati Keezhur.

This is a village situated at a distance of 5 kms from Atomic Energy station, Kudangulam. There is the Vishwamitra Mahalinga Swami temple here where he has performed the yagnas. Even today he is believed to be present there in his subtle body. There is a small well near the temple.

When the well was dug, a huge heap of ashes was found. Some scientists from abroad took samples of those ashes for investigation. They confirmed that those ashes was approximately 17,50,000 years old.

The ashes include those of the Munis killed by Tataka, those of the kings who accompanied Tataka and who were killed by Rama and Lakshmana, and even those of Tataka herself. Scholars of humanities believe those ashes to be from them. If it was otherwise, there is no chance of such a huge pile of ashes being found there.

Another proof that Rama had come to Tamil Nadu is the existence of this Vishwamitra Mahalinga temple.

Thus it is possible for miracles to take place even in Kaliyuga. We should become deserving of that. That's all. Shri Vadiraja was a very ideal devotee. He was restrained as well. He had no ego whatsoever. Perhaps that is the reason why the Lord came in search of him, is what we can understand from his life.

The Navagraha Stotra composed by Shri Vadiraja is very popular.

While undergoing education, while facing adverse effects of aspects of the nine planetary positions, or while going for a promotion, chanting the Navagraha Stotras and worshipping Shri Hayagreeva will remove all obstacles and bestow all success.

16

Navagraha Stotra composed by Shri Vadiraja

Bhasvanme Bhasayettasyam chandrashchahladkrudbhavet
Mangalo Mangalam Dadyad Budhashcha Buddhataam Dishet
Gururme Gurutaam dadhyaatkavishcha kavitaam Dishet
Shanishcha Sham Prapayatu Ketu: Ketu:jaye Arpayet ||
Rahurmeraahayedro Grahassantu karagrahaa:
Navam Navam Mamaishvaryam Dishantve Te Navagraha
Shanedinamane: Sunosvaneka Gunasanmane
Arishtam Harame Abhishtam Kurubhakuru Sankatam ||
Harehanugrahaarthaya shatrunaam nigrahaya cha
Yaadiraajayatiproktam Grahastotra Sada Patteth ||
Iti shrimadvadirajaa Pujya charanaavirachitam navagraha Stotram
Sampurnam |

17

Shri Hayagreeva's darshan to Vedanta Desikar

The place where Poigai Azhwar incarnated is said to be one among the seven places that bestow liberation namely Kancheepuram. Close to this is Tiruttanga in Thuppal where Shri Vedanta Desikar is said to have incarnated. He was born as the son to Tiruvengada Mani.

At a very young age, he learnt all the Shastras from his maternal uncle Appullar. He had an inclination in the worship of the Divine from a very early age. After the death of his maternal uncle that inclination and detachment from worldly things grew stronger.

He went to Tiruvahindapuram. He had the darshan of Shri Deivanayaka Peruman and the goddess. He then went to the Sri Narasimha Sannidhi on Oushadatri mountain and sat in front of the Sannidhi under an Ashwattha tree. Seated there he chanted the Garuda mantra taught to him by Appullar several lakh times.

One day Garuda Azhwar with a luminous body gave darshan to Shri Vedanta Desikar. He also presented him with an idol of Shri Hayagreeva and initiated him into the Shri Hayagreeva mantra.

There was no limit to the joy felt by Shri Desikar at that time. He flew in the air like a Garuda with wings. His mouth started pouring out a stream of Slokas.

He composed and sang the Garuda Panchat consisting of 52 Slokas in praise of Garuda Bhagawan and expressing his gratitude to him. It is a very enchanting composition indeed. It would not at all be an understatement to say that each of them is like a gem.

We shall look at one of them before proceeding further.

Shri Desikar says, "In this world, the Kings and Princes when they set off for war to defeat attacking enemies, they were sent off with the accompaniment of the loud sounds of several musical instruments such as the Trumpets. There would be loud cries hailing the victory of their respective leaders. Besides, young girls would sprinkle auspicious flowers etc. in the air. This was the normal practice since historical times.

Similarly, Garuda Azhwar, in order to get his mother released from slavery, went to bring elixir. His singular aim was to defeat the Devas and bring the elixir that was hidden in the Deva Loka and with that aim in mind he flew off.

His huge wings were flapping ceaselessly while en route. The sound of those flapping wings was like those of the victory sounds. The swift movement of the wind due to the strong flapping of his huge wings caused huge waves of air to move resulting in an echoing sound which was like the victory sounds made to gather people around.

When Garuda Azhwar flew in the sky, the speed of his wings shook the stars in the skies and losing their positions fell off. They came shooting down to the Earth and those shining star- fall was a real treat for the eyes.

It was comparable to the beauty of the young girls who would stand in the four directions welcoming the victorious king with their shower of auspicious flowers.

In this manner, while moving swiftly across the skies crushing the army of the Devas with his enormous flapping wings, Garuda Azhwar is also praying that he may be protected from the hellish pain that comes with it. This is the essence of the song.

Now, we shall come to incidents from his life journey.

Later, Shri Desikar chanted the Shri Hayagreeva mantra given to him by Garuda Azhwar, day and night with single pointed concentration, holding all the five senses under control. As a result of this, the ocean of knowledge and the ocean of mercy, Shri Hayagreeva Bhagwan manifested before him, giving him darshan and at that time he spit the elixir from his mouth. Due to this, Shri Desikar became proficient in studies, and his limitless knowledge, the yearning for poetry, skills in all art forms expanded like the ocean. All Shastras, Vedas, Puranas and their nuances penetrated into his mind. This has been referred to by Shri Vedanta Desikar himself in one of his Stotras.

This is an extraordinary composition consisting of 33 Slokas. The first stanza of the composition is as follows:

Jnyananandamayam Devam Nirmala sphadikakrutam
Aadharam Sarvavidhyanaam Hayagreevam Upasmahe.

We have already seen the explanation of this stanza. We shall look into another one presently and see its meaning.

The sound of the neighing of Shri Hayagreeva appears to be like the union of all the branches of Samaveda. It even leads one to contemplate as to whether it is another expression indicative of the essence of Rigveda Mantras! That's not all! His neighing sound seems to give the meaning of all Yajurveda mantras drawn to it.

It carries tremendous strength. It is capable of breaking through any obstacle and difficulty faced at the time of studies. It is like the white foam on the huge waves that rise on the ocean of knowledge. In this sense, it is the essence of Rig, Yajur and Sama Vedas. Shri Desikar praising the sound of the neighing of Shri Hayagreeva says it is an excellent illumination that is adept in removing the darkness of ignorance of other religions.

Having got the grace and blessings of the horse faced Bhagwan, all skills flowed like water in him.

Apart from being a lion in Veda and Vedangas, he was an expert in the area of Mantras and Tantras as well.

As a result of this he attracted several enemies.

Once a snake charmer challenged him and engaged him in a competition. Let us look into that story in the coming chapter.

18

The Devotee who controlled snakes

When Shri Desikar was living in Tiruvahindipuram, some students from Kancheepuram came there. They said, "Swami we have been waiting to see you and listen to your commentaries for such a long time. Please fulfill our wishes whole heartedly. Please visit Kancheepuram."

Shri Desikar too had the desire to go to Kanchipuram and serve Perarula Perumal. Therefore, he decided to use this as an opportunity. After taking permission from Tiruvahindipuram Perumal he left along with some disciples for Kancheepuram.

On reaching Kancheepuram, he straightaway entered the Perumal temple and worshipped him. He shed tears of joy. When meeting after separation, do we need to talk? He stood there speechless, words failed to come for expression; a satisfied silence ensued. He stood there totally absorbed for quite some time. He then returned to his normal awareness.

Kanchi's Perarula Perumal's beauty had stolen his heart. He writes about it in a song.

Perumal's crown shines like the brilliant Sun its rays spreading everywhere, his face is like the Moon with its shower of cool rays, he is wearing two fish shaped rings on his ears. When they move it looks like as though two fish are dancing with the intention of attacking each other.

There is a mark on his chest called the Shri Vatsam, and the Goddess also lives there forever. The stomach region of the Lord into which at the time of the great annihilation or pralaya everything gets absorbed and also from which all creation begins appears beautiful.

All the people of the world have come to surrender to him for attaining liberation and are standing there at his holy feet. Vedas are singing in praise of his body to the extent possible and his glory. Imagining this state of service to the Perumal by Vadiraja Perumal it gave the impression of a mirage in the desert.

He stood firm and tall as though even a mountain like the Attigiri Mountain would be required to bend to his ways.

He was like the beacon of light to shatter the darkness of ignorance in the world.

He is the treasure that Brahma is in search of and he is the one who is hiding within everyone as the Antaryami.

One even feels like imagining him to be the inextinguishable elixir yearned by the slaves.

Shri Desikar's heart flooded with emotions of having gained the service of such a Perarulalan.

Having immersed in the waters of Bhagawan's beauty his heart was filled with joy and in that state of bliss he returned home.

During his stay at Kancheepuram, one afternoon, a snake charmer came in search of him. He had several snakes with him. Some of them were poisonous. Others were non-poisonous ones. He showed them to Desikar.

"Sir, you are learned in Mantras and Tantras. I heard that you have the skills to subdue even poisonous creatures. Through your knowledge of mantras, can you control the poisons in my snakes?" he asked.

"Due to the grace of Devaraja my mantras have the strength and capability of subduing poisonous creatures" said Desikar.

"I too am no ordinary man. I have caught huge black cobras straight from their pits and even Nagarajas without being struck by their fangs in dense forests and have brought them in the very bags that I caught them in. Once the Chieftain of this village wrongly blamed me and put me behind bars for two days."

"I boiled with anger. I desperately wanted to take revenge on the official who had imprisoned me for no fault on my part. I went to the forests. Wandering here and there I caught hold of several varieties of snakes. Some of them were poisonous. I plucked out the poisonous teeth from their mouths."

"That night when everything had calmed down, I went to the house of that official. I threw in ten snakes through the window of his house. I came and went to sleep on a bed of hay."

"It would have been about 4 O'clock in the morning. The women from that house came running outside shouting, "Snakes! Snakes!" Their shout was music to my ears."

"On that day, wasn't I too, a falsely accused victim, I had pleaded saying that I had not done anything wrong, I cried, still that cruel minded fellow's heart did not change. I was unjustly framed with crime and imprisoned. Now that I have taken my revenge, I am very pleased."

"I could have let the snakes in the house without pulling out the poisonous teeth from the snakes. If only I had done that none in that house would have survived. But I did not like to do that."

"I thought that I too should punish him the way he did to me. I accomplished that cleverly. I have not shared what I had done with anybody else so far."

"The shouts of the members of that household in fear and panic were pleasing to me. Their cries and screaming could be heard to the other corner of the street. I slipped away unseen."

The snake charmer ended his story with great pride.

He continued, "Swami, I heard people in this town that you have the knowledge of some Garuda Mantra. I am a snake charmer. I have several snakes with me. I shall let them loose. Can you tie them up with your mantras? If you do that I shall proclaim before all that you are truly a very great man!"

Shri Desikar refused to have any kind of competition.

"Don't be afraid. I just want you to say those mantras and control these snakes of mine and that is enough for me" assured the snake charmer, a little reassuring at the same time a little teasingly.

Shri Desikar had been listening to what he said with a smile. He opened his basket. There were several snakes with yellow, white, wheatish and black colors.

He poured them out on the floor.

"Swami, from now on you should not hesitate. You are always having the protection of Shri Hayagreeva. Please participate in the competition" said his friends encouragingly.

The snakes started sliding on the floor and dangerously running all over the place. Shri Desikar drew some lines on the floor. The snakes were unable to cross those lines. They wrinkled there itself.

One Nagaraja crossed the lines. It angrily pounced towards Shri Desikar. He immediately chanted the Garuda Mantra. Instantly Garuda appeared in the skies from nowhere and picking up all the snakes, flew off.

Nobody expected that. Due to such a sudden turn of events, the snake charmer shuffled. If his question had contained defeat in itself, that was one part, but on the other he had lost even the snakes which was his very source of livelihood. This affected him greatly.

Realizing his folly, he said, "Sir, I fully accept that you are an expert in Mantra and Tantras. It was on these snakes that I earned a living and on which my family was sustained. I was getting at least a one- time meal with what I earned from them. Therefore, please have mercy and get them back for me. I shall not forget this favor until death" he begged.

Shri Desikar too felt pity on the snake charmer's condition. Immediately he created and sang the Garuda Dandaka sloka. The next moment, Garuda brought back the snakes taken away by him and dropped them down.

The snake charmer was very happy. He said, "Swami, you have definitely proved that you are a master of all skills". Saying this humbly, he bowed down and gathering his snakes left the place.

In this manner Shri Vedanta Desikar humbled the pride of a snake charmer and demonstrated his mountain like prowess in Mantra Shakti. Just as the mountain, though huge and forbidding, it is calm and cheerful, so also Shri Desikar was a very calm, humble person and conducted his life in a very simple manner.

19

The White horse came in search of Desikar

Having lived for a long time in Kancheepuram, Shri Desikar had the intense desire to have the darshan of Shri Ranganayakar. He decided to visit Tiruvarangam. One day he left for Tiruvarangam and when he reached Tirukkovalangur, it was late in the night.

He looked for a place to spend the night. He found an empty portico of a house which was that of a businessman dealing in groundnuts. He sat down and performed the daily puja to the idol of Perumal which he had carried along with him along with all the necessary materials, without committing on anything. However he had no Naivedya. Since there was no alternative, he requested to the deity, "O God, you understand my condition. Therefore today I can offer you only water as Naivedya, please accept it." In this manner he concluded the pooja and he too partook of the water as Prasad. Thinking of the Lord, he lay down to sleep.

In a short while, due to the fatigue of travel, he was fast asleep.

It was midnight when he heard voices calling out, "Swami, Swami, wake up!"

Shri Desikar opened his eyes. Before him stood the groundnut dealer businessmen, a little frightened and in a sleepy mood.

Shri Desikar looked at him questioningly.

"Swami, a white horse has entered our warehouse of ground-nuts and is eating the groundnuts. I tried to drive it away several times, but it does not seem to budge. I am afraid, can you please come Swami?" said the businessman.

Shri Desikar closed his eyes and went into meditation.

Aha! This is the leela of the very gracious Paramatman, he realized.

"Do not be afraid. Today I had left my Perumal to go hungry. He has entered the warehouse with hunger. What can be said of his supreme grace!" he said.

"Swami, I didn't understand anything. You left Perumal hungry, you say?"

"You will not understand. Please bring me some milk" said Desikar.

He immediately went and returned with a glass of milk.

He offered that to the horse in whose form Shri Hayagreeva had given darshan, as Naivedya.

The very next moment the mysterious horse vanished just as mysteriously as it had come.

"What a surprise!" said the businessman.

When he came to know that the horse that had come to his house was Shri Hayagreeva himself, his joy knew no bounds. Since the person who was the reason for this was Shri Desikar, he took him as his Acharya and bowed down to him several times. His prosperity increased several fold. Since then he started serving Shri Vedanta Desikar and Shri Perumal. In this manner, Shri Hayagreeva made known the glory of one his favorite devotees, Shri Vedanta Desikar to the world.

20

Podhigai Muni Agastya

Shri Hayagreeva is the source or origin of all Learning, Skills, and subjects like spirituality; he is the fountain head and store-house for all knowledge. He is the eighteenth incarnation of the Tirumal.

Tirumal is considered as the Supreme by the Vaishnavites, Parashakti is considered as the Supreme Goddess by the Shaaktas, between whom he is considered as the connecting bridge. It was he who instructed the Shri Lalitobhagyanam and the Shri Lalita Sahasranamam to Agastya Muni.

Agastya was a stalwart in the Tamil language. He is one among the Maharishis. He has enormous powers. He was born not from a woman's womb but form a mud pot. We can call him the Test tube baby of those ancient times.

Once in the distance past, Mitra and Varuna, went for a stroll and happened to move through Indra's abode, Urvasi, the heavenly dancer arrived there. When both of them saw her they wanted to get intimate with her and enjoy the pleasures of being close to her. As a result of this the semen dropped from their bodies. They gathered this in a pot and it was from this that Agastya and Vasishtha were born. Since Agastya was born from the pot or Kumbha he is also called Kumbha Muni.

There was an objection for Aryans to cross beyond the Vindhya Mountains. The first person to boldly retaliate against this objection and cross over was Agastya. He came from the North to the South and corrected many of the practices prevalent there.

When the marriage of the princess, daughter of the Mountain King was to take place, Devas and Munis rolled over to go there and be a witness on the occasion, as a result of which the Meru Mountain sank and the south rose up. The Gods, when they saw this said, "You alone could do this to make the earth balanced. Therefore you go to the South and remain there."

He too immediately got ready to leave. Several Arya princes too got ready to accompany him. While on their way southwards, he approached Ganga and requested her to give him Kaveri river.

Then he went to Jamatagni Muni and asked his son Tiranadhumagni to be given to him as his student. When he put forth the proposal to ask for his sister Lopamudra in marriage, he agreed to it too. In this manner getting married to Lopamudra he reached the Vindhya Mountains. Those Mountains stood tall and refused to allow them to cross over. He cut down its pride and making it a flat land he proceeded on with his journey.

May Vatapi get digested!

In the Vindhya forests, there were two Asura brothers by the name of Ilvalan and Vatapi who were causing immense trouble to the Munis. Any Muni or Rishi coming to the forests were being tormented by them with their Maya Shakti and they had made it their habit to kill them for food.

When Agastya Muni arrived there, Ilvalan and Vatapi converted themselves into a shepherd and goat respectively and welcomed all of them. The shepherd very humbly said to Agastya, "O Mahamuni! We are pleased to welcome you here! Please accept the meals that I offer you today" in a show of false humility.

Agastya too agreed very readily.

Immediately Ilvalan, the shepherd, killed his brother Vatapi, the goat, cooked it and offered it to Agastya. He too ate it to satisfaction.

After that, Ilvalan called out to his brother, "Vatapi, come out"

Vatapi desperately tried to tear the stomach of Agastya and come outside. This was their usual practice of killing the Munis who came there. But his time they had not come across an ordinary Muni, but Kumbha Muni, one whom Shiva Himself had sent to the South because of his prowess and ability.

Agastya rubbed on his stomach and said, "Vatapi Jeeranodbhava". Vatapi was completely digested in the stomach. Agastya then reduced Ilvalan to ashes through his yogic powers. In this manner the two Asuras who were killing innocent Munis as though like child's play, also faced death in the same playful manner in the hands of Agastya Muni. Play is dangerous was the lesson that the Asuras learnt the hard way.

He then proceed to Siyagiri where a river rose dangerously spreading its waters and then without being of use to anyone, it joined the ocean. He, who had realized that the use of corn is as food, the use of stone is as a statue, so also realizing that the waters of the river is life giving to the people, brought the waters from river Ganga and purified this river.

Later, with the assistance of the young princes he had brought along with him, directed the course of flow of the river to one side and allowed it to flow through the country side. This led to increase in productivity and business and also provided drinking water in the places which faced shortage. That river was the Kaveri river, which is often addressed as the hen that gave golden eggs. From there, he continued his journey towards Tiruvenkadu. After having the darshan of Venkata he arrived at Podhigay Mountain and established his ashram there where he nurtured his disciples with loving care.

21

Agastya's surprising wedding

Shri Hayagreeva is the origin, source and sustainer of all education, skills, principles, spirituality, all kinds of norms, and learning. He is the eighteenth incarnation of the Tirumal.

Tirumal is considered as the Supreme by the Vaishnavites, Parashakti is considered as the Supreme Goddess by the Shaaktas, between whom he is considered as the connecting bridge. It was he who instructed the Shri Lalitobhagyanam and the Shri Lalita Sahasranamam to Agastya Muni.

Once while navigating through the Cosmos through the power of his mind and yogic skills, Agastya Muni went to the Mountain peaks of the Himalayas for Tapas. There he found several Munis and Rishis engaged in penance standing upside down and seeing them he was surprised.

He approached them and asked, "Munis, who are you? Who are you looking at and meditating upon in this pouring snow, standing upside down?"

We are fully realized Munis; in our clan, a Mahamuni by the name of Agastya has been born on the Earth. He is not getting married and is observing strict Brahmacharya. That is totally contradictory to the nature of other people from his land. He should get married and experience the joys and sorrows; that is the order of the Lord. Since he is wandering freely as a Sanyasi, the sorrows that he is supposed to experience, we as his ancestors are experiencing them in this manner.

Agastya was shocked on hearing this.

"You are asking about our welfare with so much concern. May we know who are you?" they asked.

"I am that Tamil Muni Agastya. I came here to do penance. O Munis, please forgive me. You are suffering because of me. I shall no longer remain standing, watching you suffer."

"I shall immediately go and finding a suitable girl, get married and engage in worldly life." He fell at their feet and prayed.

The Munis were happy. They blessed him saying, "Friend, you will get a wife to your liking". Later, their misery having been cleansed returned to Pitruloka.

Agastya started searching for the girl whose was destined to be his wife in all the three worlds. He wanted a girl who would be submissive to him and also not be an obstruction in his observance of Brahmacharya and accordingly he looked for such a girl in the Indra Loka and Chandra Loka but could not find.

One day he went to Satya Loka and encountered Brahma. He saw next to him Vishnumaya in a beautiful feminine form. His eyes and intention settled on her for a moment. He then returned to the Earth.

As this was going on, a King by the name of Kaveran in the Vidarbha region, was ruling his Kingdom leading a happy life along with his wife. The couple had an unfulfilled desire. They did not have the joy of bearing a child. In spite of observing several vows, visiting various pilgrimage centers, performing innumerable Homams, they were unable to fulfill that desire.

In the end Kaveran and his wife began intense Tapas to Lord Shiva. As a result of the tapas, Lord Shiva manifested before them. He said, "Kavera, there is no child destined in your life this life time. Do not exert yourself unnecessarily. Give up penance and rule your kingdom well." Saying this he disappeared.

Kavera and his wife were dejected. When Lord Shiva himself had said that they would not bear a child this lifetime, then whom could they go to for lamenting their fate. They cried bitterly. After some days, they consoled themselves and started leading a normal life. Years passed by. Their youth vanished and old age set in.

Old couple get a young child

Under those circumstances, Agastya Muni came in search of the couple to the Vidharbha region. The aged couple, Kavera and his wife welcomed him enthusiastically and respectfully attended to him.

They surrendered at his feet. Closing his eyes for a moment, Agastya went into meditation and understood the reason for their sad state of heart and mind.

With a smile, he blessed them, "May you be blessed with a child."

Even though the couple were happy on hearing this, they felt within themselves, "Time has passed by, we have become old. Will we be able to bear a child now? Lord Shiva himself has said, that we are not destined to have a child" they looked at the Muni doubtfully and with hesitation.

With God's grace there is nothing impossible. A dead tree can grow leaves, a dry well can spring with water, most certainly. Therefore through my yogic powers I shall bring a child for you. Consider her your own child and bring her up with love and care. When she reaches the appropriate age, I, myself shall come and marry her.

The joy of the couple knew no bounds. When God gives, he breaks open the skies and showers his blessings. Is this the same thing?

"Even without our asking, Agastya Muni comes in search of our palace and finding us blesses us with the joy of a child. There is no more sorrow for us. Pleasant days have come into our lives at last," they rejoiced.

Agastya stood chanting Veda mantras with both hands extended in front. Through his yogic powers, Vishnumaya whom he had seen that very day in Brahma Loka manifested as a small child in his hands.

The delicate flower like girl child that he held in his hands opened her toothless mouth and was laughing away as he handed her over to the couple who gently put her in a cloth cradle and stood there watching her, their happiness reaching the skies.

They bowed down several times with humility and thanked him profusely.

The Gods, when they came to know of this came down to the Earth to have a look at the child. The child had all the 64 virtues befitting a perfect girl and was extremely beautiful. Therefore they named her Lopamudra. The name signifies possessing all the sixty four skills.

The child started growing rapidly in height and size. She was a divine child, was she not? Her every movement was graceful and pleasant to look at. Her smile drowned them in joy. They addressed her as Kaveri.

The palace which was in darkness for several years appeared to have suddenly been lit by a crore Suns and the life of Kavera Maharaja seems to have suddenly transformed overnight. There are no words to describe their happiness, proving even destiny wrong, they thanked Agastya Muni again and again for blessing them with a girl child.

They brought her up with utmost care. There were several maids to cradle her, sing lullaby to her, to feed her with milk, and take care of her in every way. Still Kavera's wife took great pleasure in taking personal care of the child. Even though she had not given birth to the child, still she was the child who had delivered her from the stigma of being barren.

As a means of expressing gratitude, even though she was the queen of the land, she gave all the motherly love to the child. Listening to her childish blabber was music to their ears. The use of ears itself is for listening to the childish talk is it not, the husband and wife said to each other and felt some pride in it too.

The child started crawling. In spite of there being several nurses around, those aged parents themselves took care of the child. They ran after her to catch her.

The nurses said, "Mother, we shall look after her. Do you need to run at this age?"

"This is our good fortune. Mahavishnu on hearing his name called, when an elephant screamed when death stared in its face as a crocodile held its leg, he immediately climbed on his vehicle, Garuda and came to his rescue and killed the crocodile. Do you remember the story of Gajendra Moksha?"

"If he wished he could have continued to lay on the Sesha naag and thrown the Sudarshan chakra from there itself. Instead of doing that he immediately climbed on to Garuda and flew to the banks of the lake. It was only after arriving there he used the Sudarshan chakra. Killing the crocodile he saved Gajendra, the reason being affection. It is that affection alone, that in spite of my advanced age, I feel like doing each and every thing for the child disregarding the inconveniences whatsoever" said the queen.

Understanding the hidden love behind the actions of the queen, everyone were very happy.

The child began picking up things that came on her way as she crawled on the floor and put them into her mouth.

Immediately she sent out instructions to the nurses to clean the floor. Worrying that the knees of the young girl would get scratched while crawling on the floor, she spread soft carpet on the floor in several places in the palace rooms.

Arrangements were made to see that there was one girl always with the child to pick up things she pointed at and give it to her.

When Kaveri started getting up on her feet and walking hesitatingly, both the King and the queen watched her intently and inwardly rejoiced at the sight. Their lives that had almost come to a halt for so long seems to have just started to get up and walk.

Leading, touching, grabbing, and feeding the rice mixed with ghee to the child was a real task; she would spill it all over herself; she would half drink and half spill the milk from its container; the mess that she kept creating all the time were watched by them with great amusement.

When the King used to have his lunch, he used to be served twenty two varieties of dishes in a huge plate, each of which was of a different color and taste. Kaveri would arrive there dragging herself. She would call him "Pappa Pappa!" The King would forget himself when she called him like that. She would come flip flap on her tiny feet near the King and put her hand into his plate.

The queen would lovingly object her.

The King would chide her and allow her to take whatever she wanted.

Swaying gently, the child would pick up what appealed to her with her left hand and laughingly put it into her mouth and chewed on it.

The taste of food, pungent or sour, was new to her. So she squirmed and made faces when confronted with different tastes. All those different expressions were a source of immense joy to the King and the queen.

The King would run after Kaveri forgetting his age and its limitations. He would want to lift her up. But his hands used to pain if he lifted her for a long time.

He used to then remember the days when he used to carry heavy iron swords and spears and it had never pained him then, but now those very hands had weakened. He used to be annoyed that even a girl as light as a flower was painful for him to life or carry.

Years passed by in this manner. Ever since Kaveri had arrived, the kingdom became prosperous. There were plentiful rains. The fields yielded good crops; grams crop yield was more than normal. The Kingdom was free from disturbances from animals, diseases and enemies and so the people were happy.

The King's challenging time

When she was seven years old, one day there was a visitor to the palace. His name was Shri Saryanandanaadar; he was a worshipper of Sri Vidya.

He requested the King, "Sir, I wish to perform the Chaturmaas Vrat for the welfare of the world. Please give a small place within your palace where I can stay and also would like to have an assistant to assist me in the puja activities."

Although on the one hand the King was happy that a great person had visited his palace, on the other he was afraid because the visitor was a short tempered man. There was no difficulty in setting up a dwelling place for him but to find a suitable assistant for him was a problem.

If there was any shortcoming in the assistance provided for his puja, he would immediately curse everyone altogether. Therefore the King appeared a little worried.

He or his wife would willingly do anything necessary for him. But neither of them were in a position to be that active and agile considering their advanced age. This question tormented the King.

Understanding her father's worry, Kaveri asked, "Appa, what is your reason for worry? Please tell me."

"You are too small, there is no use telling all these things to you," said the King.

"Appa! Even a small needle is enough to pick the tooth, is it not? Tell me without any fuss!" insisted Kaveri.

"The Muni who has come to stay at out palace is going to perform puja for a whole month. I couldn't get an obedient person for his assistance. Me or your mother could do it but being aged we can't do all the running around at the allotted time so properly."

"Is there no one in our palace to do the work?"

"There are thousands of people who can do the job. But to do it to his satisfaction is a little difficult. Even a small thing not done properly will annoy him and he could curse all of us. I am not able to find a proper solution. That is the struggle that we are facing" said the King.

"Is that all? Let go all worries! Instead of you, I myself shall do all his work to his satisfaction and earn a good name too" said Kaveri.

"No Child, he is a short-tempered man!" said her mother with a little anxiety.

"Amma, haven't you said that —where anger is there, there alone is true virtue? That would be applicable to him as well is it not? Leaving aside all other Kings, he has come in search of our palace, that itself goes a long way in showing how much love and respect he has for us."

"I have been born to you after a prolonged period of time. That must be known to him. Therefore even if I do not come up to his expectations he should not mind. Besides, I shall be all eyes and ears to help him in his puja; I shall not give him any scope for complaint." Kaveri spoke confidently against their argument and gave them the confidence.

They too agreed. Kaveri took two of her friends and going to the ashram met the Maharishi. She did namaskar and said, "Swami, I have come to help you in your puja work."

Having already known her, the Maharishi said, "Come child!" He looked at her lovingly and placing a hand on her head blessed her. "Young lady, for your age, you are more mature, more self-confident and have a great sense of service. May you lead a healthy life."

22

The history of Shri Lalita Sahasranamam

Kaveri assisted the Maharishi by picking the necessary flowers for the puja, preparing the Naivedhya, removing the old flowers, cleaning the puja vessels shining and bright and such other work.

The puja for the whole month was carried out very well. Before leaving the palace the Maharishi called Kaveri and instructed her the Shri Vidya mantra.

"Young girl! If you perform the puja with devotion chanting this mantra with full faith, you will be blessed with all kinds of prosperity. You will get the yogic powers to assume whichever form you want and to go to whichever place you desire." He said and left.

Since that day, Kaveri started chanting the Shri Vidya mantra with reverential fear and devotion. As a result of that she derived various kinds of benefits. She became extremely knowledgeable, she acquired all kinds of Siddhis. By then she attained the age of sixteen.

Marriage concluded

Kaveri grew up to be a beautifully matured girl as though like the third phase of the Moon increasing its crescent to attain the stature of a Full Moon, striking all with her splendor and beauty.

Can a daughter of a King be married to any ordinary man? Will she be able to give up all the luxury and fineness of a palace? Will she be able to live in the forest with ordinary clothes? Many people were confounded with these questions.

"Amma! It was Agastya Muni who asked you both to take care of me, is it not? When I attain maturity, I should be given in marriage to him, he said, is it not? Then, when you had already accepted it, would it be right for you to object to it? It would be like going against your word which is wrong. Father, you are the King of a country. If you behave like this then it will become a precedent for your people to go against truth. Therefore you don't worry. Wherever I may be, I will always be happy" said Kaveri assuring.

Having attained some satisfaction with her reply, the King and the queen completed the marriage rituals in a befitting manner. Agastya took Kaveri and visited several pilgrimage centers. After having the darshan of the Lord at all these place they returned to the ashram at Kancheepuram.

He performed the daily puja to Kamakshi Amman as per the Shri Hayagreeva Shri Vidya Upasana rituals in a very proper manner. Shri Vidya japa, Shri Lalita Sahasranama archana and Trisathi with the three hundred names, Aradhana etc used to be performed at the end of which Agastya Muni would make his wife Lopamudra herself seated as a representation of Kamakshi Amman and perform her puja and conclude the daily rituals. This was carried on for several years.

To witness the puja performed by Hayagreeva to Kamakshi Amman, and participate in it, the thirty three crores of gods and goddesses and the King of Gods, Indra used to come to Kancheepuram.

One day, Agastya Muni went to Kancheepuram for having the darshan of Kamakshi Amman. At that time, the Devas met him and said, "Agastya Muni! You are so blessed! Do you know that your wife is participating daily in the Sri Vidya puja performed by Shri Hayagreeva?

Shri Hayagreeva looks at her as Shri Kamakshi Devi and performs her puja. Lopamudra too is accepting it and giving her blessings."

Agastya Muni did not believe it. "My wife does not leave me and go anywhere. Therefore you contention that she is coming to Kancheepuram daily cannot be true" he said.

"No Agastya Muni! We are telling you what we saw with our own eyes. At the end of the puja when the Manai palagai, a wooden Aasan is placed, Lopamudra comes flying from somewhere and gladly accepts the puja and after receiving it she disappears. This happens daily. We have seen the event happening even today and we are returning from there," said Indra, the King of the Devas.

"O Devendra! Seeing someone else like my wife you are saying it is Lopamudra. From the day of marriage to me she has not left me for even a single minute and gone anywhere."

Indra replied, "If you don't believe us, then you yourself go to the Sri Vidya puja one day and see for yourself."

The very next day Agastya Muni went to the Suhasini puja performed by Shri Hayagreeva. At the end of the puja when the Manai was placed, Lopamudra appeared there mysteriously and sat down. She accepted the Gulamrutam offered by Shri Hayagreeva at the end of the puja and after taking a little of it, she returned the remaining and he too consumed it with reverential devotion and offered it to the others present there.

Agastya looked at the girl intently. How astonishing! He couldn't believe his eyes! She was his wife Lopamudra herself.

How is that possible? Only if she has attained the eight Siddhis it is possible for her to appear from air and manifest for a short while and disappear into thin air again. If she has to attain those Siddhis, it would take several years of penance and practice of Yoga. He did not remember her having done that even for a single day. He was perplexed.

Sri Vidya Upasana

On returning to the ashram, he asked his wife, "Was it you who came to the Suhasini puja of Shri Hayagreeva and received the Naivedyam?"

"Yes, Swami".

"How did you get these Siddhis, which is available only to very great Yogis and Tapasvis? I have not seen you do Japa or Tapas even for a single day!" he asked with surprise.

"When I was seven years old, a Mahamuni had come to stay at our palace. I was the assistant for his pujas during his stay. Pleased with me, he instructed me into the Sri Vidya mantra. I practiced it very intensely. I got these Siddhis as a result of that. Travelling to the desired place and returning became very easy" she said.

The Sri Vidya mantra is an Aryan Treasure. If that has to be attained as a Siddhi, one has to have earned merits for several life times. After performing several hundred pujas to Mother Abhirami, one becomes deserving of her grace. You have received that grace."

"I have heard that Sri Vidya mantra among all the mantras, bestows several kinds of yogas. I have also heard that it bestows all kinds of Siddhis even without any Japa or Tapa. When I saw that happen through you I was surprised. Devi, will you please instruct me in that mantra" requested Shri Agastya Muni.

"A wife instructing her husband is against the Shastras. Besides, she is subservient to me and so you asking that from me casually is also a possibility. Above all that, to instruct you into the mantra, verily that supreme Shri Hayagreeva himself has come to Kancheepuram. This is Kamakshi Amman's command given by herself so go and have his darshan" said Kaveri.

Some days passed by. One day, she looked at Agastya Muni and asked, "Did you seek the instruction?".

"No, there was too much crowd there. In that crowd, I could not go near Hayagreeva. After everybody did namaskar, he tell s them all to be seated. I could not go near him and speak to him" said Agastya.

"It is Ambika's orders that only after instructing you that he should give up this body and go to Vaikuntha. Therefore do not postpone it further. Tomorrow when you go to the puja, even after everybody has sat down, you remain standing. Then his vision will fall upon you. Why are you standing? He will ask. Say that Lopamudra sent me here. Then he will take care of you." She guided him and sent him the next day.

The next day Agastya did as he was told. "Why are you standing Agastya?" said Shri Hayagreeva. "I have been waiting for you all these days. I would have instructed you and gone to Vaikuntha. Anyway, I shall begin from today" saying this, he started the teaching.

In this manner, he taught the Shri Lalitobhagyanam, and Shri Lalita Sahasranamam for the benefit of mankind so that they may evolve and attaining salvation. After instructing this he left for Vaikuntha.

In this manner, Hayagreeva Perumal, was also the guru of Agastya Muni and has instructed him in a very astonishing manner and given him Mantra upadesam. There is no doubt that praying to him will bring knowledge and wisdom in large measure.

23

The Kshetras where Hayagreeva has manifested

There are several places where Shri Hayagreeva manifested and where temples of worship have been built. Among them the most important one is the temple at Tiruvahindipuram.

Muvaragiya oruvanai Muvulagu Undupizhndu Alandane
Devar danavar Chendru Chrndiraincha Tantiruvayindipurattu
Mevu jyotiya velvalavan Kalikandri Viritturaitta
Pavudandamihppattivai Paadida pavangal payilave.
Periyatirumozhi – 3110

This was the devotional charter created by Tirumangai Azhwar at Divyadesam which is about 3 km away from Cuddalore.

Main deity - Deyvanagan - The deity is standing facing the East. He is also addressed as Devanathan.

Procession- Among the three one is Idevan.

Mother - Vaikunthanayaki - Hemambhuja Vallitthayar is also addressed as Bhargavi.

The Sesha Teertha, and Garuda Teertha has now become Ketila Teertha.

Vimanam - Chandra Vimanam, Shuddha Sva Vimanam

Garuda, Adisesha and Shiva are among those who have had the darshan.

Growth

Once an intense war ensued between the Devas and Asuras. The Asuras were gaining an upper hand in the battle. The Devas approached Tirumal (Mahavishnu) and surrendering at his feet, prayed to him to save them. Shri Narayan mounted on his Garuda and fought the war on behalf of the Devas. The Asuras opposed him also vehemently. With determination Shri Narayan set off his Sudarshan chakra and destroyed all the Asuras.

During this war, Shiva came to assist the Asuras. So, to defend the Sudarshan chakra, the Trishul was used. But the Trishul, unable to destroy the chakra, went and stood beside it as though in protection of it. When Shiva saw the scene through his Divine vision, the Supreme presented him with the vision of the Trinity to Shiva. He sent the Trishul back to Shiva. At the request of the Devas a temple was built at that holy spot. That holy place is the Tiruvahindirapuram Divyadesam.

Perumal here is depicted with four faces and carrying the conch and chakra.

Due to the exertion at the war, Perumal too had felt thirsty. He asked for water. Garuda immediately went flying in the air to bring water for the Lord. Adi Sesha hit his tail hard on the Earth which split open and from the depth a fountain flew up and brought the water. Adi Sesha handed over this water to the Lord and thereby his thirst was quenched.

Since the fountain manifested through the opening in the Earth split by Adi Sesha, this Teerth was called Tiruvagindupuram. In the course of time this became Tiruvayindipuram.

The Teerth here is named after Adi Sesha and is called Sesha Teertham.

Uniqueness

Adi Sesha split the Earth open and brought forth a spring of water from within. Garuda went through air and brought water from the Viraja river. In this manner this place is where the two vehicles of Mahavishnu, Adishesha and Garuda brought water for the Lord.

The water which was brought by Garuda flows here as Garuda Azhwar Teertha. With the passage of time it dried up. Later it got transformed into the present Ketila river.

Garuda prayed to Mahavishnu, to accept the waters that he had brought too. Bhagwan accepted his request. Due to that during the Annual Rathotsav a puja is performed on the banks of the River Ketila also.

The Viman here is just like that at Vaikuntha where in the Shuddha Sattwa Viman, beneath it. To the East is Mahavishnu, to the South is Dakshinamoorthy, to the West is Narasimha and to the North is Brahma.

The pujas are performed here as per the Vaikana agamas. This place also has a history of being the place of incarnation of Shri Sriniva of Tirupati as well.

The incarnation of an amsa of Mahavishnu as Lakshmi Hayagreeva took place adjacent to the sanctum of this temple itself.

The master of all learning, Hayagreeva, is present here in the form of an idol with a white horse faced human body wearing yellow robes, holding the five weapons, and as though pushing the nectar of the Vedas as foam from the mouth, grace bestowing eyes, embracing the great goddess in his heart. Just in front of the Sannidhi of Deyvanayaka, on a slightly elevated position is the place called as Oushadagiri which is very ancient and filled with extraordinary powers. There are 74 steps here which are representative of the 74 Simhasanadhipatis created by Shri Ramanuja according to elders.

It was in this place that Garuda Azhwar instructed the Moola mantra of Hayagreeva to Shri Vedanta Desikar. The Garuda here is seen standing with hands folded, an unprecedented manifestation.

This is the holy place where Shri Vedanta Desikar chanted the Hayagreeva mantra and was blessed with the darshan of Shri

Hayagreeva personally. Shri Desikar lived here for 40 years in a house built by himself where he is also said to have dug a well with his own hands. The house where he lived is present even today.

Why did he dig a well? There is an interesting story behind it.

The well dug by Desikar

When he was staying at Tiruvahindipuram he used to worship the Perumal daily which made the people of the area jealous. One among them came there. One day he approached Desikar and said, "Swami, the whole community considers you an expert in all skills which they say was bestowed upon you by Shri Ranganayaki Thaayaar herself."

"I didn't believe that; you should have the necessary potential if you are to truly attain those capabilities. The equation will be settled only if you demonstrate that to me" he argued.

Desikar normally ignored such crazy challenges. But his friends and well wishers requested him to accept the challenge and defeat the questioner. Only if they are approached in this manner, they will stop disturbing with these unnecessary enquiries. This will also put an end to such wasteful argumentations, they insisted.

Shri Desikar too acceded to their request and accepted the challenge. The man said, "Swami, I am a construction worker. I build wells very well. I want you to build a well with the bricks that I give you. That's all" he said deceptively with a smile.

Desikar accepted it with a smile. The competition began.

The man started giving him crooked and broken bricks purposely. It is possible to set the bricks around the circular well beautifully only if they are of a proper size. However this man, intent upon defeating Desikar, was offering only very irregular bricks. The crowd which was watching this were perturbed and worried as to what would happen.

But Desikar, receiving the bricks handed over to him by the man, instead of objecting or refusing it, with his experience and above all due to the blessings of Kanchi Bhagwan, he used the bricks skillfully and built a beautiful well. When he was done constructing the well, every one praised Desikar and clapped their hands.

The construction worker, seeing this, fell at his feet. He said, "Swami, forgive me. I was arrogant that I knew everything and that is why I behaved in this manner. I was selecting only useless bricks and handing them over to you. But you were so skilled and artistic in placing the bricks that you have constructed this well in a grand manner. As far as I know, I have not met such a clever constructor all my life. The pride that I had in my skills has been squashed."

"This skill has not come to you as a family heritage. Truly, it is the gift bestowed upon you by the Sarveshwara. I accept that." He praised Desikar profusely and left. The well that he had constructed is there even today. The idol of Shri Hayagreeva whom he worshipped is still there in the Devanatha Sannidhi in the temple at the foothills.

If we serve the Lord...

Do you worry that however much you earn, there seems to be no relief from the burden of debt? Are you concerned that you are never free of illness whatever medicines you may take? There is no need for worry at all. Just go once and have the darshan of Perumal and your troubles will vanish like a whiff of cotton.

Even those who wanted to get relieved from the cycle of birth and death and those who live with the dejection of not wanting to have a birth anymore and are just pulling on with their lives, can also go to Tiruvahindipuram can, after having the darshan of Devanathan, see spring return to their lives.

Students studying in schools and colleges can see progress in their studies by way of better marks if they go and do service of Hayagreeva at Tiruvahindipuram . Interest in studies will increase. Hindrances will go away. Memory will improve.

For securing better marks

Students who are poor in their studies, or are facing some obstacles in their learning and understanding the lessons can go to this place and pray to Hayagreeva. They can offer pen, notebooks, pencils, book or honey and after placing them at his feet, they can take them back. A garland of cardamom should be offered to Hayagreeva and a puja is performed after putting the garland on him. After the puja a bit of the honey should be rubbed on the tongue and a cardamom from the garland if eaten, one will receive all his blessings. The knowledge and intellectual sharpness will increase day by day as stated by the priest at the temple.

The Teertham or holy water offered as Prasad here is very unique. It is related to the Divine. It is the Teertham that was worshipped by Shri Vedanta Desikar. If we consume this Teerth, all sicknesses are believed to go away.

The horse's mouth is continuously flowing with water. The same is true of Shri Hayagreeva too. If the elixir flowing from his mouth is tasted, all shortcomings will go away and life will become sweet.

During the Vedic period, the Asuras did very heinous crimes as a result of which they earned an unbearable burden of sins. Unable to bear the consequences, they lost their houses, they lost their land, and with hunger and sickness haunting them they suffered a lot. They then went and prayed to Shri Hayagreeva. They sang his praise and earned the nectar from his mouth. As a result all their sins were washed away and their lives turned around for the better.

At Tiruvayindapuram, the Lakshmi Teertham is offered which is also a herbal water. There is no doubt about it as it is close to the elixir from the mouth of Shri Hayagreeva.

Those who have sung in praise of Perumal

Tirumangai Azhwar alone has sung the glory of this place in ten poems.

Shri Vedanta Desikar has sung the Morning three O'clock wake up song for the Perumal.

The garland of pearls composed by Shri Vedanta Desikar is as follows:

Manjulavu Cholai Chuzha Yindai Mannucheer
Varaiyeduttu Neerai Alitta maachil Vasudevane
Chencholanpar Chindai Kondu Teetilaada Dootanai

Terumoorndu Desuyarnda Selvam Deyva nayaka
Vecholaalar kaalattur Veeshu Paasam Vandenmel
Vizhundamundi Yaanarndu Veezhvadarkumunna Nee
Anja Lanja lanja lendralikka Vendumacchuda
Adiyavarkku Maruliyarkku Madiyavarkku Meyyane.

This is the sacred place where great Munis lived and blessed with their auspicious deeds. In the language of North India there is the Devanayaka Panchat and Achyuta Shatam in Prakritik language sings the glory of this place.

In the Pillai Perumal Iyengar 108 Tirupati Antadi, it is written:

Anbaninda chintataiyaraya Aainda Malartoovi
Munpaninda Neer enakku Moouthiyare –Enbar
Yemyindirapurattarkku Inrodundaraanaar
Talamaiyindira Purattar Taan.

He has sung in praise of this place in these words.

Among all the 108 divine places sung by the Azhwars, this is the only place where Shri Hayagreevar is having a separate Sannidhi where he is seen giving blessings to all seated here. This is the uniqueness of this place. Perhaps it is for this reason that Shri Vedanta Desikar came here and did penance chanting the Garuda mantra and through him got the instruction of the Shri Hayagreeva mantra and chanting that mantra got his darshan as well. Besides, he also got the water from his mouth as a result of which, extraordinary skills emerged out of him and flowed. He lived as an embodiment of all skills and knowledge.

Here the sannidhi is open from 8:30 to 11:30 in the morning and between 4:30 and 7:30 in the afternoon. The most important day for Shri Hayagreeva is Tiruvonam and therefore on that day and the Thursday of every week, special pujas are performed here.

Other Places where Shri Hayagreeva manifested

The next place is Tiru Indalur, Mayapuram. Here, in the Parimala Ranganatha Swami temple, on the expanse in the loft there is a very old Hayagreevar Sannidhi. Here both Shri Vedanta Desikar and Hayagreeva have graced the place.

In the bigger Sri Rangam temple in front of the Thaayar Sannidhi, in the Desikar Sanniddhi, there is an idol of Shri Hayagreeva.

Shri Hayagreeva had instructed the Sri Lalita Sahasranamam to Agastya Muni. As though to substantiate this, the Kamakshi Amman temple is situated right in front of it and contains the statues of both Agastya and Hayagreeva.

In Nanganallur in Chennai, there is a separate temple for Shri Hayagreeva Peruman.

In the ashram of Shrirangam, Lakshmi Hayagreeva is gracefully seated for worship. In the Tiruvallikkeni Vyasa's Mutt, and at the Vedanta Desikar's temple at Mayilai, Shri Hayagreeva has manifested as a bestower of blessings on his devotees.

The idol of Shri Hayagreeva at the Mysore Parakala Mutt which was worshiped by Shri Vedanta Desikar is still being worshipped and pujas are still being performed there.

Next to the Punnai Nallur Tanjavur, Punnai Mariyamman temple, is the Mandapam housing the chariot of Kodanda Rama Swami temple. There is a separate sannidhi of Hayagreeva here.

On the Pondicherry- Dindivanam-Pondicherry highway, there is a village called Morattandi , in the Mahapratyankara temple, there is a separate sannidhi of Shri Hayagreeva. All facilities are available here.

In Chennai's Medavakkam, in the Srinivasa Peruman temple on top of a small hill, there is an idol of Shri Hayagreeva.

Near Chitrakulam in Tirumailai in Chennai, in the Shrinivasa Perumal temple, at Shri Vedanta Desikar's sannidhi Shri Hayagreeva's idol is locating blessing devotees.

In Chennai's Villivakkam, next to the Soumya Damodara Perumal temple there is a prayer hall for Shri Hayagreeva. The hall was constructed by a devotee out of his immense affection and devotion to Shri Vedanta Desikar. Shri Hayagreevar is seen gracing the place and blessing the devotees.

In Chennai, West Mambalam, next to Ayodhya Mandapam, is the Satyanarayana Perumal temple and the Adi Keshava Perumal temple, one can receive the blessings of Shri Hayagreeva and have his darshan.

Similarly Hayagreeva can be worshipped at the Chennai Nandambakkam Kodandarama Swami temple and Srinivasa temples.

In the smaller Kancheepuram village there is the Atisonpettai Kulam where there is the Vilakkadi temple. In the same street are the Tuppul Vedanta Desikar temple and Deepa Prakashar temple. In the Desikar Sannidhi Lakshmi Hayagreeva statue can be found. Adjacent to the temple is the Shri Parakala Swami Mutt where also Shri Lakshmi Hayagreeva is granting darshan and can be worshipped. Shri Hayagreeva is worshipped in the Varadaraja Sannidhi at Kancheepuram as well.

24

To gain victory

In a separate temple in the upper Kaveri, in Kumbakonam, Shri Hayagreeva can be seen with Mahalakshmi seated on his lap victoriously. Therefore, as a symbol of love and grace he grants darshan as Shri Lakshmi Hayagreeva. If he is worshipped with a single minded devotion, education will improve, fear of failures will go away, one will secure good marks and knowledge will increase.

On the days of Ashwini and Mula stars, if Shri Hayagreeva is clothed in yellow robes and worshipped with prayers all skills will come searching for the devotee.

On the banks of the river Kaveri, he is seen seated facing the North and is very powerful. Performing his puja here is enough for students to attain proficiency in education. Offering a garland of cardamom on Thursdays will transform even dullards to get good marks and attain success.

On every Tiruvonam day of the month, the Moola mantra Homam is performed to Shri Hayagreeva in a grand manner. If one participates in this Homam ceremony, soulfully offer your prayers, and then chant his Moola mantra 9 or 27 times, one will definitely find progress in one's studies is the belief of many students.

Therefore, school and college students come in swarms to attend the Shri Hayagreeva Moola Mantra Homam in this temple and pray. Sometimes one can see the queue of students standing for worship extend right up to the street.

The students worship Shri Hayagreeva by placing pen, pencil, notebooks, Hall tickets etc. at His feet and taking them back.

So, students who want to attain success and emerge victorious in your studies, should go to the Kumbakonam Upper Kaveri and receive Perumal's grace and blessings.

The Slokas that gives strength to the hands

All of us desire victory. But sometimes, victory seems to be far-fetched. In such times, our skills and efforts alone are not enough it is necessary to have Divine blessings. Chant the following sloka and worship Shri Hayagreeva with total devotion. One will get strength in one's hands.

Chandramandala Madhyastam Hayagreevam Sunirmalam
Jnyana Mudrataram Devam Shankha chakradharam Vibhum
Pustakam Vamahassethu Dharinam Vanamalinam
Kreedahaarakeyura Katakaadhyair alankrutam.

For Educational development

Clean the photo of Hayagreeva, apply Kumkum and turmeric paste, and on every Punarpoosa nakshatra day offer a garland of Marigold flowers, chant the Hayagreeva Stotra with devotion 11 times, there will an improvement in studies. There will be greater yearning. Marks will improve. Lighting a lamp with ghee and offering milk as Naivedhyam daily will bring better results.

The 4th and 5th house on the horoscope are the houses for education. If these are afflicted then the person may not be good in studies. It is for such students that Shri Hayagreeva is waiting to bless. Pray the following sloka:

Gnyananandamayam Devam
Nirmala Sphatikaakrutam
Aadharam Sarva Vidyanam
Shri Hayagreeva Upasmahe.

Chanting the above sloka will open up the fountain-heads that were closed to studies. What could not be understood earlier will start giving new meaning. One will be meritorious in studies and start securing higher marks in exams.

Shri Hayagreeva is the very embodiment of all knowledge, bliss and light, shining like the brilliance of white marble and is the support for all arts and skills. It is to him that I worship. This is the meaning of the sloka.

His horse face is shining like the brilliant Sun. He is four armed. Besides he is granting blessings along with Mother Lakshmi. He is seen with his hand showing the mudra of granting boons. He protects from danger with his hand showing the Abhaya mudra thereby granting fearlessness; he is also seen as a yogi with a tuft of hair on the head; thus Shri Hayagreeva grants us darshan in various ways as seen in the different temples.

Students undergoing education should meditate upon him for overcoming obstacles in their studies. If they chant the Hayagreeva Gayatri daily, and please him one will be blessed with unparalleled benefits.

Hayagreeva mantras

Students who are weak in their studies, or those who would like to pursue music, dance and such other fine arts and who wish to attain proficiency in the same should pray to the ocean of knowledge Shri Hayagreeva and worship him.

Some children are not able to speak fluently, they stammer. If such people and even those students who complain of poor memory worship Shri Hayagreeva, they will be relieved of their shortcomings and achieve progress in their lives.

According to astrology, those who are under the influence of the transit period of Mercury and Moon and those who are under the influence of the Lords of the 4th and 9th House should perform the Abhishekh of Hayagreeva on the day of Tiruvonam nakshatra, perform his aarti and offer a garland of cardamom. Their sorrows will be removed, and they will be filled with enlightenment. The problems in studies will go away.

Om Vageeshwaraya Vidmahe
Hayagreevaya Dheemahi
Tanno Hamsa prachodayat.

This is the Hayagreeva Gayatri. His Moola mantra is as follows:

Utgeeta Pranavotgeeta Sarva Vageeshwareshwara
Sarva Vedamaya Chintya Sarvam Bhodaya Bhodaya.

While chanting these slokas, and while listening to others, the vibrations created out of these help in acquiring single pointedness and will assist in the widening of higher knowledge, and improvement in their physical and mental health.

Chantng these mantras daily, focus on studies will improve, students' inclination towards their studies will increase, those working in schools and colleges will also find relief from problems in their lives. Shortcomings faced in pursuing higher education will disappear.

There are no rules and conditions for the chanting of the Shri Hayagreeva murthy Gayatri mantra or the Jnyanandamayam Devam sloka. Students and children can chant the mantras as and when they find time. Praying whole-heartedly while chanting the mantras will bring untold benefits to the devotee.

25

108 Names of Shri Hayagreeva

1.   Om Hayagreevaya Namaha
2.   Om Mahavishnave Namaha
3.   Om Keshavaya Namaha
4.   Om Madhusoodanaya Namaha
5.   Om Govindaya Namaha
6.   Om Pundarikakshaya Namaha
7.   Om Vishnave Namaha
8.   Om Vishvambharaya Namaha
9.   Om Haraye Namaha
10. Om Adityaya Namaha
11. Om Sarvavageeshaya Namaha
12. Om Sarvaadharaya Namaha
13. Om Sanatanaya Namaha
14. Om Niradharaya Namaha
15. Om Nirakaraya Namaha
16. Om Nireesaya Namaha
17. Om Nirupadravaya Namaha
18. Om Niranjanaya Namaha
19. Om Nishkalankaya Namaha
20. Om Nityatruptaya Namaha

21. Om Niramayaya Namaha
22. Om Chidanandaya Namaha
23. Om Sakshnine Namaha
24. Om Sharanyaya Namaha
25. Om Sarvadayakaya Namaha
26. Om Shrimate Namaha
27. Om Lokatrayadheeshaya Namaha
28. Om Shivaya Namaha
29. Om Saaraswata Pradaya Namaha
30. Om Vedotdhaytre Namaha
31. Om Vedanidhaye Namaha
32. Om Vedavedyaya Namaha
33. Om Puratanaya Namaha
34. Om Purnaya Namaha
35. Om Purayitre Namaha
36. Om Punyaya Namaha
37. Om Punyakeertaye Namaha
38. Om Paraatparasmay Namaha
39. Om Paramatmane Namaha
40. Om Parasmai Jyotishe Namaha
41. Om Pareshaya Namaha
42. Om Paarakaya Namaha
43. Om Parasmai Namaha
44. Om Sakalonishatvedyaya Namaha
45. Om Nishkalaya Namaha
46. Om Sarvashastrakrute Namaha
47. Om Akshamala Jnyanamudra Yuktahastaya Namaha
48. Om Varapradaya Namaha
49. Om Purana Purushaya Namaha
50. Om Sreshtaya Namaha
51. Om Sharanyaya Namaha
52. Om Parameshwaraya Namaha
53. Om Shantyaya Namaha
54. Om Dantaya Namaha
55. Om Jitakrodhaya Namaha
56. Om Jitamitraya Namaha

57. Om Jaganmayaya Namaha
58. Om Jaramrutyuharaya Namaha
59. Om Jivaya Namaha
60. Om Jayadaya Namaha
61. Om Jatyanasataya Namaha
62. Om Japapriyaya Namaha
63. Om Japastutyaya Namaha
64. Om Japakrute Namaha
65. Om Priyakrute Namaha
66. Om Prabhave Namaha
67. Om Vimalaya Namaha
68. Om Vishwarupaya Namaha
69. Om Vishwagoptre Namaha
70. Om Vidhistutaya Namaha
71. Om Vidhaye Namaha
72. Om Vishnawe Namaha
73. Om Shivastutyaya Namaha
74. Om Shantidaya Namaha
75. Om Shavanti Parakaya Namaha
76. Om Shreya Pradaya Namaha
77. Om Shrutimayaya Namaha
78. Om Shreyasaam Padaye Namaha
79. Om Ishwaraya Namaha
80. Om Achyutaya Namaha
81. Om Ananda Rupaya Namaha
82. Om Pranadaya Namaha
83. Om Prithvipataye Namaha
84. Om Avyaktaya Namaha
85. Om Vyakta Rupaya Namaha
86. Om Sarvasakshine Namaha
87. Om Tamoharaya Namaha
88. Om Ajnyana Nashakaya Namaha
89. Om Jnyanine Namaha
90. Om Purnachandra Samaprabhaya Namaha
91. Om Jnyanadaya Namaha
92. Om Vakpataye Namaha

93. Om Yogine Namaha
94. Om Yogeeshaya Namaha
95. Om Sarvakamadaya Namaha
96. Om Mahamounine Namaha
97. Om Mahayogine Namaha
98. Om Mouneeshaya Namaha
99. Om Shreyasamnidaye Namaha
100. Om Hamsaya Namaha
101. Om Parama Hamsaya Namaha
102. Om Vishwagoptre Namaha
103. Om Viraje Namaha
104. Om Swaraje Namaha
105. OM Shuddha Sphatika Shankashaya Namaha
106. Om Jatamandala Samyutaya Namaha
107. Om Adimadhyantarahitaya Namaha
108. Om Sarva Vageeshwareshwaraya Namaha

Shri Lakshmi Hayagreeva Pancharatnam

Jnyaanaanandamalaatma Kalikalushamahar
Toola Vatoola naama
Seemadidaatma Bhuma Mama Hayavadanaa
Devata Daavitaari:
Yata Shwetaabhja Madhyam Pravimala Kamala
Sraktaraa dugdaraashi
Smeraa Saa Raaja Raaja Prabhruti anutdhiipadam
Sampadam Samvidattaam   1

Tara Taradhinatha Sphatikamani Sutaa
Heera Haraabhi Rama
Rama Ratnabhdhi Kanyaa Kushali Kusha
Pariramba Smarambha Danya
Manyanandyaarhadaasya Pranatati
Pritraana Straatha Deeksha
Daksha Sakshat Krutaishaa sapati Hayamukhi
Devata Sa Avataan Na: 2

Antardhwantasya Kalyam Nigama Hrudasura
Dhwamsa Naikanta Kalyam
Kalyanaanaam Gunaanaam Jaladi mabhinamat
Bandhavam Saindhavasyam
Shubhramashu Praajamaanam Datata Maridarou
Pustakam Hastaganjai
Patraam Vyagyana Mutramapi Hrudi Sharnam
Yaamyutaaram Sataram.   3

Vande Tam Devamadhyam Nama Tamaramahaa
Ratna Koteera Kotee
Vatee Niryatna Niryat Krunikana
Masruneebuda Paadaamshujaatakam
Shrimat Ramanujarya Shruti Shrikaraguru
Brahma Tantra Svatantrai
Pujyam Prajyam Sapajyam Kaliripu Gurubhi

Sarva Dashvottamangam. 4

Vidya Hrudya Anevatya Yatanaga
Karunasaara Saara Prasaaraat
Dheeraadhaara Dharaaya Majani Janimaataam
Taapa Nirvaapayitree
Shri Krishna Brahma Tantraadima Pada kalijat
Samyameendraarchitam Tat
Shrimad Taamaadhibhuma Pratayatu Kushalam
Shri Hayagreeva Naama 5

Shrimat Vadiraja Swami's
Shri Hayagreeva Stuti

1. Lasad̄asya hayagr̄iva lasadoshthadvaȳaruna
   Lasaddant̄aval̄i'sobha hayagr̄ivalasatsmita
2. Lasatph̄ala hayagr̄iva lasatkuntalamastaka
   Lasatkarn. a hayagr̄iva lasannayanapa nkaja
3. Lasadv̄iks.a hayagr̄iva lasadbhumandaladvaya
   Lasadgr̄iva hayagr̄iva lasaddhastalasadbhuja
4. Lasatp̄ar'sva lasatprstha kaksam sayugasundara
   Hayagr̄iva lasadvaksah stanamadhyavalitraya
5. Hayagr̄iva lasatkukse lasadromalāancita
   Hayagr̄iva lasann̄abhe lasatkatiyuḡantara
6. Lasad̄uro hayagr̄iva lasajj̄anuyugaprabha
   Hayagr̄iva lasajjanḡayugma p̄ad̄ambujadvaya
7. Hayagr̄iva lasatp̄adatalarekh̄arunadyute
   Lasannakh̄a ngul̄isobha hayagr̄iv̄atisundara
8. Lasatkir̄ita keȳura kankan̄a ngadakundala
   Hayagr̄iva lasadratnah̄arakaustubhamandana
9. Hayagr̄iva lasanmadhya lasacchandanacarcita
   Lasadratnamaȳakalpa sr̄ivatsakrtabh̄ushan
10. Hayagr̄iva lasatk̄anchiratnakinkinimekhala
    Hayagr̄iva lasadvastra maninupuramandita
11. Hayagr̄ivendubimbastha lasachankhakshapustaka
    Lasanmudra hayagr̄iva lasadindusamadyute
12. Hayagr̄iva ram̄ahastaratnakumbhasrtamrta
    Hayagr̄iva samana'sr̄icaturupopasevita
13. Hayagr̄iva surasreshtha hayagr̄iva surapriya
    Hayagr̄iva suraradhya jay'sishtajayeshtada
14. Hayagr̄iva mahavīrya Hayagr̄iva mahabala
    Hayagr̄iva mahadhairya jatadushtavinashtida
15. Bhayam mrutyum kshayam vyarthavyam.
    nanamayam cha me
    Hare samhara daityare hare narahare yatha

16. Bhaktim shaktim viraktim cha bhuktim muktim
    cha yuktida
    Hare me dehi daityare hare narahare yatha
17. Sada sarveshtalabhaya sarvanishthanivrttaye
    Hayagrīvastutih pathya vadirajayatīrita
18. Cintamanir Hayagrīvo vaseyasyanishevitah.
    Sopi sarvarthado nrunam kimutasau hayananah.
      Iti ´srı Hayagrīvastutih. samaptam

Shri Lakshmi Hayagreeva Sahastra Namavali

Om Shri Hayagreevaya Namah
Om Shreem Namaha
Om Hamsaya Namaha
Om Ham Hayagreevaya Namah
Om Jamomatmate Namah
Om Kleematmatmane Namaha
Om Shriya Shriyai Namaha
Om Shri Vibhushayanaya Namaha
Om Parojase Namaha
Om Parabrahmane Namaha
Om Purbhuvasuvaradhimaya Namah
Om Bhasvate Namaha
Om Bhagaya Namaha
Om Bhagavate Namaha
Om Svastyatmane Namaha
Om Svaahaatmane Namaha
Om Nama Atmane Namaha
Om Svatatmane Namaha
Om Sroushatatmane Namaha
Om Alamatmane Namaha
Om Voushatatmane Namaha
Om Hum Phat Atmane Namaha
Om Humatmane Namaha
Om Hrim Namaha
Om Krom Namaha
Om Hloum Namaha
Om Yatatata Namaha
Om Kalka Krivaya Namaha
Om Kalanathaya Namaha
Om Kamadaya Namaha

26

Goddess Saraswati over the ages

Goddess Saraswati is one of the three main female goddesses worshipped by the Hindu religion. Saraswati is the Goddess of Education, Lakshmi is the goddess of prosperity and Parashakti is the goddess of courage as per the Puranas and Itihasas.

Goddess Saraswati is the authority over learning. Rigveda speaks of Saraswati as having originated as a river on the Earth. Saraswati means, knowledge, fame, and enlightenment and therefore it is represented by the white color and ignorance is depicted as darkness. This is the reason why Goddess Saraswati is seen seated on a white lotus and wearing a white sari. There is a raga by the name of Saraswati.

Kanda Puran says that goddess of the arts resides in the tongue of all human beings. This is so not only for the people of this country but for the rest of the world as well. Goddess Saraswati is also addressed as Shruti Devi and Vak Devi. The Jains call her Jina Aishwarya as is found in several of their texts. Aputtiran gets the Akshaya paatram from the god Chinta Devi. That god is Saraswati Devi herself according to Manimekalai kavyam.

The Buddhist religion celebrates Goddess Saraswati. She is also addressed as Mahasaraswati, Aryasaraswati, Vajraveena Saraswati,

Vajra Sharada, and Vajra Saraswati. This goes to show that she is a deity who is beyond all religions.

Saraswati

Buddhism has introduced several Hindu deities in various ways. The Kings favoured these Divine aspects of the Supreme and celebrated then during their reign. This also helped in bringing the people under one protective umbrella and eliminating religious and racial conflicts.

Although this may be going on one side, the descriptions in the Smritis about the Hindu gods being super human also greatly fascinated them. Not having a desire only for the progress of their states, but also desired with the help of the Divine blessings of the gods, to reach their expected state of progress and prosperity. They searched for a lot of Gurus for this purpose. Pundits who had done well in their schooling and education and, who had gained good knowledge and wisdom through experience found top positions in King's palace.

The glory and energy of each Gods and Goddesses were explained to the Kings in detail. They started praying and worshipping the gods for protecting their lineage, meeting their needs, guidance for the path of their states, and removing their fear.

Saraswati (6th century sandstone)

There is nothing surprising in the fact that the extraordinary play and Leelas of the Gods and goddesses impressed the Kings very much. The various things done by them as a means of pleasing them have also appeared in random essays from time to time. In this manner, ancient stories and literary works, arose enormously.

Since the Kings and their officials believed those stories more than necessary, within a short time, the faith in Gods became an inherent part of the Kingdom and way of life itself. This is one of the reasons why those divine stories did not die out even till the present days. In the Buddhist religion, the Shinto sect have accepted them for centuries after centuries, celebrated them and worshipped them with faith and devotion.

Saraswati's worship in Japan

We can see worship of Goddess Saraswati in Japan as well. One can get to see a methodical worship of the Hindu goddess Saraswati there. Among the Buddhists in Japan, there is a worship to a female deity by the name of Benzaidin. This was brought to Japan by some merchants from India during the period between the 6th and 8th century.

This goddess is said to have emerged from a Sutra named the Golden Light and from whom language came into existence. She is painted in gold and is seen seated on a white lotus holding a Biva a traditional Japanese flute in one hand. This reminds of the Veena held by our goddess Saraswati. This female deity is common to Buddhists and Shinto sects.

Saraswati can be seen to have been worshipped by the Romans as Minerva and by Greeks as Athena as is evident from their literature. Even today Saraswati, depicted with three faces, six hands and called as Manchushree is being worshipped by the Buddhists. Jains worship Mahasaraswati representing the sixteen arts.

27

Stories about Goddess Saraswati from the Puranas

Matsya Purana describes the birth of Saraswati as follows.

When Brahma was engrossed in deep meditation for a prolonged period of time before the beginning of Creation, his body got divided into two, one portion of which was male and the other portion was female. The female was Goddess Saraswati. Along with her, Brahma created Manu. The rest of mankind were created from Manu.

There is a similar story about Brahma. When Brahma started the work of Creation, from his tongue emerged the goddess of speech, the Vakdevi, Saraswati.

In another story, Saraswati, whose father was Brahma, emerged from his forehead. As soon as she manifested, Brahma got attracted towards her. When Saraswati objected to him as it was improper for him to approach her in this manner as she was his daughter, still, for some reason, Brahma did not change his stance. His eyes pursued her and followed her.

Accordingly, in every direction he grew a head. When she disappeared into the sky, Brahma grew a fifth head grew facing upwards into the sky.

Shiva, Vishnu and the other Devas tried all they could to prevent this insatiable craving of Brahma. Still, he did not pay any heed to them. He stood firm on getting married to Saraswati. Since there seemed to be no other way out, they consented to it.

Still, since he got married without heeding to the words of Gods, they cursed him that he shall not be worshipped on Earth. This is the reason for there being no temple for Brahma or his being worshipped anywhere on Earth.

Saraswati Devi, is being worshipped due to her own glory as the goddess of learning. She does not get any glory from her husband.

Saraswati Devi and the Trimurti

Once, Andhak, son of Kashyap Rishi, was caught stealing the Parijat tree from the heavens and while bringing it down to the Earth.

The Trimurti, Brahma, Vishnu and Mahesh got together to decide as to what should be the punishment to be given to him. At that time, since their Shaktis too were present, they manifested in three feminine forms in red, white and black colors. The white form was that of Saraswati, red was that of Mahalakshmi and black was that of Mahakali.

Antiquity of River Saraswati

Several stories appear in the Puranas regarding the river Saraswati.

Once, an unresolved enmity arose between Rishi Vishwamitra and Rishi Vasishth. As a result, Rishi Vishwamitra, who had Kshatriya origins, decided to completely finish of Sage Vasishth. He had River Saraswati to assist him in this deed.

Saraswati lamented as to whether she was being used to kill Vasishth. She feared that in retaliation she might be cursed. So she agreed to assist him out of fear.

Rishi Vishwamitra asked her that, when Sage Vasishth was asleep, she was to bring him to Vishwamitra somehow or the other. That was all. Saraswati agreed to that.

Yet, her heart did not permit in her being an accomplice in the killing of a Brahmin. So, she went to Sage Vasishth and told him of the treacherous scheme of Vishwamitra and in turn asked him, "O Maharishi, please tell me as to what I should do now. I shall do as you say" saying which she stood there in all humility and obedience.

Vasishth said, "As per his command, you go for me. Let what has to happen, happen."

She gathered sage Vasishth as a flower and took him across. The Muni too consented to it. When she neared Vishwamitra's ashram, Vishwamitra rushed angrily outside with his axe, intending to kill Vasishth.

Seeing this, Saraswati got frightened, and deciding that she should not become a party to this sin, she sprang forth for the Patal Loka taking Vasishth along with her.

Seeing this act, the enraged Vishwamitra cursed, "Your waters will be turned into blood, you leapt to the Patala and therefore this will result in your vanishing from everyone's sight."

Since that moment, river Saraswati disappeared from everyone's sight and began to flow like a river of blood and expanded on all sides. This was amusing to the Asuras. They drank the blood of the river that flowed into the Patala Loka and drinking it in ample measure increased their strength enormously.

Several years later, some Munis arrived there. Seeing Saraswati river flow as a river of blood instead of flowing as a holy river, they felt pained. They saw through Divine vision in meditation as to what had happened. In order that she might attain her Divinity they did penance to Mahavishnu. Realizing that this could be possible only at the Triveni Sangam, they got the three rivers, Ganga, Yamuna, and Saraswati to come together in one place.

This is how the Triveni Sangam at Allahabad came into existence. After that, the Asuras dipped into the waters of the holy river and got all their sins washed off and attained Salvation. There is another story similar to this one.

Once, the Asuras grabbed away the palm leaf manuscripts and disappeared. When she appeared in the form of a river on the plains of Daneshwar, this incident took place. Ashamed with the incident, she leapt into the Patal and hid herself from the sight of everyone. Later, at the prayers from the Munis, she once again came on the Earth at Prayag at the Triveni Sangam.

In the Aadhi parva of the Mahabharata, there is some information in relation to Saraswati Devi. A great monk by the name of Madinara did a yagna on the banks of the river Saraswati for twelve long years. At the end of the yagna, river Saraswati granted him the darshan in the form of a beautiful woman. The woman entered into conjugal relations with the monk as a result of which a child was born. The child's name was Dhansu. His lineage prospered. It was in that lineage that Shantanu was born who later got married to Ganga and had many children.

In this manner, there are several stories related to Saraswati which can be found in our ancient literary works. Why did she turn into a river? We shall presently look into that aspect.

28

The Divine yearnings of the goddess

The Rigveda speaks of the Goddess flowing as the Saraswati river. The word Saras means, light, fame and ceaseless flowing. Allowing the arts to flow without inhibition and leading one to the heights of fame and glory is her essential nature and that is why Slokas are sung in praise of Saraswati Devi.

Why did she become a river? Let us get to know about that as well.

Once there was a prolonged war between the Devas and Asuras. The Devas were on the verge of defeat. Therefore, in order that their main weapons may not be snatched away, they went to Muni Dadeechi and handed them over to him for safe keeping. He too agreed to the arrangement.

The Devas then hid themselves somewhere, in fear of death. Somehow, Vruttrasur searched them out and invited them for battle. Immediately, they approached Muni Dadeechi and requested him to return their weapons.

He replied, "You handed over the weapons to me and disappeared for an indefinitely long period of time. Being responsible for taking care of them, I reduced them to ashes and drank it."

The Devas were devastated. They all said together, "O Muni! What shall we do now?"

"Indra and Devas, do not panic. I have the ability to die whenever I want. Therefore I am prepared to give up my life for your victory. On my spine I carry the powers of all your weapons. You can take that and prepare a weapon with it. Vruttrasur had asked that his death cannot be caused by any weapon made of metal. To kill him, a weapon made of the bones of my spine will be useful." Saying this Muni Dadeechi gave up his life.

Indra got a Vajarayudha made from the bones of Muni Dadeechi. With this weapon he killed Vruttrasur.

At the same time, Dadeechi's wife was pregnant and was due for delivery. She gave birth to a beautiful boy. She was distressed over her husband having given up his life for the sake of the Devas. She wished to give up her life too. She prayed to the Vanadevi in the forest to take care of her child and left it in the shades of a banyan tree leaving the roots to take care of it and she too climbed on to the funeral pyre.

The banyan tree took care of the child. His name was Peepalata.

When he grew up, under the impression that the Gods had killed his father, he was filled with anger. He was desperate to take revenge. Receiving the blessings of Brahma he undertook rigorous penance to Shiva.

One day, Shiva manifested before him. He said, "I shall open my third eye. If you have the strength and capacity to bear its force, then I shall give you the boon you ask for."

He too agreed to it. The moment Shiva opened his third eye, Peepalata shuddered, unable to bear the heat. He continued to do more rigorous penance to increase his strength. Again when Shiva opened his third eye, he could not bear the heat. He once again did intense Tapas and accumulated enormous powers.

Seeing his relentless efforts, Shiva was pleased with Peepalata. He manifested before him and said, "Peepalata, you are struggling to gain victory in the work undertaken by you. I shall grant you a boon, ask what you wish for. Along with that I also give you the choice of opening my third eye as well."

Peepalat opened the third eye of Shiva. Instantly a bigger fire shot out from it. He gave it to Peepalat saying that "it is very unique. It has more heat as compared to its size. It is capable of destroying the whole world. Therefore use it very carefully." Saying this he vanished. There are people in the North who worship Peepalata, who opened Shiva's third eye, as an incarnation of Shiva himself.

Having got a weapon that is indestructible by anyone, he takes it and goes after the Devas to destroy them. They ran frightened. They hid themselves in Patal Loka and lived there. He followed them there as well.

They surrender to Brahma. They ask him that Peepalat be told of all that had happened.

When Peepalat reached Brahma Loka, Brahma explained to him, "Dadeechi Muni was not killed by the Devas. He himself willingly gave up his life in order to make his spine available for making the Vajrayudha to make a weapon to kill Vruttrasur."

Even after hearing this his anger did not subside.

Brahma said, "Peepalata, I shall bring your father from Swargga Loka by the Pushpak vimaan. You can directly ask him about it."

Dadeechi arrived there in the Pushpak Vimaan. Peepalat's mother also came with him. They spoke to him consolingly.

Dadeechi said, "I had given up my life in order to save the Devas. But you are bent upon destroying them. This is wrong. It is totally in contrast to my service and sacrifice for them. Therefore give up your feelings for revenge." Dadeechi tried to make him understand.

Peepalat was consoled by these words.

Peepalat's anger subsided. But what was to be done with the ball of fire? Where was it to be kept? Each one gave his own suggestion. Where is that thing in the world that can bear the intensity of its heat?

Just then, the Fire itself made an astral announcement. "Put the ball of fire in a golden pot and consign it to the ocean. I shall remain there by the name of Vadamukha Agni. I shall get the necessary refuge there. I shall not cause any harm to anyone."

Putting the ball of fire in a golden pot, Brahma gave it to Saraswati and asked her to take it. He asked her to take the form of a river and take the pot and assign it to the ocean.

But, unable to bear the heat of the fire, she struggled. Therefore, Brahma asked, Ganga, Yamuna, Tapi and other river goddesses to get the work accomplished.

All of them together went and taking the pot they placed it safely at the bottom of the sea bed. The place where the pot was first given to Saraswati is the Tapta Kund in Badrinath as it is known presently.

29

She is seated on a white lotus

Wearing a white silk sari, and seated on a white lotus, the Goddess of arts, has the swan as her vehicle. She is striking a sweet sound on the chord of her Veena she holds in her hands. One hand holds a rosary and the other a book. She is the master of all arts and indicative of the need for education she holds a book in her hands. She is a genius in fine arts, still there is no limits to learning. Therefore one should continue to learn one's whole life and to demonstrate that, she holds a book in her hands.

We can never see another female goddess known for her sacrifice as she. She is said to have done penance on the tip of a needle so to say, to get married to her husband Brahmadeva according to the stories in the Puranas. There are no temples separately for her. The reason being she is believed to dwell on the tongue of everyone who is engaged in studies and learning and that itself is considered to be her temple and manifesting there she gives her blessings.

She has a rosary in one hand which is called as Akshar mala. In the other hand she is seen holding a book. She holds the Veena with her two hands in the front. The Akshara mala is symbolic of spirituality and the manuscripts that of knowledge. The Veena chords are representative of the 64 arts.

The Akshara Mala in her hands has beads equal to the number of letters in the Northern language namely fifty one. Therefore this is indicative of the language. The Northern language is considered as the father and the Tamil language is considered as the mother. In that respect, Goddess Saraswati is the origin of the Norther language and the sustainer and flourisher of the Tamil language. There is no poet who has not sung her praise, there is no poet who has not worshipped her.

Her vehicle is the swan. The swan is one bird that has the capability of separating the milk from a mixture of milk and water and drinking only the milk. In the same manner, those who are educated are able to discriminate between the good and the bad and have the wisdom to select only the good. This is a unique distinction of education.

Apart from bestowing the great wealth of education on man, which enables him to procure victory and stature, she secures for him great respects of other learned persons and Goddess Shri Saraswati makes the accomplishment of this possible. She is deserving of the pride of being addressed as Vak Devi. Worshipping Goddess Saraswati will bring knowledge and success. Her benevolent glance can make even a dumb person to pour forth poetry from his mouth. There are several instances in proof of this.

She, who is Brahma's wife, is knowledge. It is a necessity not only for children alone. People of all ages can benefit from not only education but also the wisdom gained through experience. In this world, every day brings a new challenge before everyone. This is an indisputable truth. The problems, the challenges that come a person faces can be met only if he has the adequate education and wisdom to handle them.

Education is not only knowledge that is obtained by reading books in schools and colleges. That is learnt knowledge. It is mere bookish knowledge. This knowledge is useful only for gathering information about the prevailing times. Equipped with information, handling life's difficulties requires a different capacity. One who bestows such subtle knowledge is Goddess Saraswati.

The knowledge that is acquired through education is bookish knowledge. It should be connected to the world. Otherwise what is it's use? In the modern times, there are still several people who are merely informed and do not yet have the wisdom of the world at all.

The fallen zucchini (gourd) cannot be useful for curry, is it not? Even if one has read hundreds of books if he does not have practical knowledge and experience he will either face failure, or he will face humiliation. In this connection, there is an interesting story that our Tamil Veteral, U V Swaminatha Iyer narrates very amusingly. Read the story of a dry Pundit who had good knowledge of grammar but had no knowledge about the world and reality of the people resulting in confusion.

30

Giants of Grammar

Tamil Grandfather writes:

To the North East of Kumbakonam, on the banks of the river Kaveri, there is a village called Karuppur. There, another Mutt owned by Tiruppanandal Kashi Mutt is functioning. In that Mutt, some scholars and Pundits who are associated with Tiruvaaduturai Mutt, are engaged in teaching and learning the Sanskrit and Tamil languages . Research in Tamil and publication of grammar books was being undertaken on a grand scale.

There was a huge dry well in front of the Mutt. There was no wall around it. The cart drivers used to drive the bullocks belonging to the Mutt, and allow them to drink the water and bring them back.

One day when I had halted in that place, a student happened to come there. He was studying the Sanskrit language and grammar from the pundits there. It was also usual to learn Tamil poems. He came running panting with fright and said that an animal had fallen into the well.

When we heard that, we assumed that one of the bullocks of the Mutt had fallen into that dry well. We rushed to the well to see. We could not find anything having fallen into the well. No water bubbles appeared either.

"The cows of the Mutt were huge, is it not? If any one of them were to fall in the well, then at least one of their horns or head would have been visible, is it not?" said one among them.

"The well is huge, water is also much. So, the cow might have fallen and drowned" said another.

"The cow falling too is not a big issue; the bigger problem is to get it out" said a third person, worriedly.

By now, several people had gathered there. The cart drivers ran here and there in panic as not knowing whose bullock had fallen in the well.

We did not know what to do. Just then, a person by the name of Deyvashikamani Iyer, looking at the student who gave us the information, "You said nothing is seen in the well" and said, "I can see something in into the well."

We all looked intently. At that time, a small chameleon was struggling to climb up the wall of the well.

He said, what can be seen there is a chameleon.

The student said, "that is what I told you."

The gentleman could not control his anger at that! He gave one hard slap on the face of that student. He said, "You Fool! You made so many of us to panic unnecessarily. The way you said, it seemed as though a bullock from the Mutt had fallen into the well. Thinking it to be so, we were all shocked."

"Had we not known the facts, in a short while two of us would have tied ropes around and got into the well. Was all this necessary at night fall? So long you have been hanging around like a smashed tamarind, now you are pointing towards a chameleon?" he blasted out.

But, the student, not taking much cognizance of the hard slap of the elderly person on his face, said, "Is the chameleon not an animal" and ran into the Mutt. He brought the classified dictionary and showed that chameleon is shown under the category of animals.

Hearing this, Iyer got all the more angry. You are a distilled fool. Throw that Dictionary into the well. If he would have said that a chameleon had fallen into the well then all this anxiety and fear could have been avoided.

Hey Grammar stalwart! Does anyone call a chameleon an animal in ordinary parlance? Have you heard it being said like that? Is it enough to digest the classified dictionary alone? Is it not necessary to know reality in the world as well?" he asked in anger.

The people standing there laughed at the nature of that educated foolish student. Some others consoled Iyer and took him away from the place. This is what the Pitamaha of Tamil literature has narrated.

Therefore, it is not sufficient only to be educated, it is also necessary to know the worldly practices. If not, the education will only be a subject of ridicule.

If there is wisdom along with education, one can shine in the world. In order attain that wisdom, we should worship at the feet of Goddess Saraswati. Our ancestors have praised such education and have written about it in the literary works. Let us get to know a little more about them.

31

The glory of education

A King alone is considered the highest he ideal person in a nation'and among its people. But a learned scholar gets the highest respect and honour than even the Kings , says Auvaiyar.

Mannanum Masara Katronai seer thookkin
Mannanin Katron sirappudayan
Mannanukku Tan desam Allal sirappalla katronkku sendravidum
ellam sirappu.

The King may not be appreciated nor celebrated by the people of neighboring countries. But, if it is known that a learned man from even an enemy country has arrived, then he will be welcomed by all and well treated. They will enjoy conversing with him. Educated people will always be respectfully entertained wherever they go.

Tamil Nadu's excellence in education

A man's place of birth and the country of birth is his own place and own country. But for an educated man it is not so. Whichever place he may visit, people will welcome him willingly like their own relatives. Whichever nation he may go to, he will be honored by the elders of the area and will always be around him. When education is capable of giving such pride, why should a person suffer without education until his death, says Tiruvalluvar, is surprising to him.

Yadanum Nadamal Uramal en oruvan
Sandunayum kalladavaru.

There are eyes on everyone's face. In spite of having eyes, if you do not have the vision then will life be beautiful? Certainly not! Similarly, everyone may have eyes, but it is education that is the benefit by the eyesight. The eyes that do not give the benefit are merely sores.
Tiruvalluvar writes:

Kannudayar enbavar katror mugattirandu
Punnudaiyar kalladavar.

If there is one thing that man has to do his whole lifetime, then that is education. Even if a person engages in studies from his birth till death, his education will not be complete; that is how vast and boundless is the ocean of knowledge. There is a saying that goes: What we know is just a fistful of sand while that which is yet to be known is as vast as the endless sand on the sea shore.
Even though education may be difficult in the beginning, it becomes more interesting later on. Kumaraguru sings:

Todangunm kaal tunbamai inbam payakkum
Madam kondru arivu agatrum.

Ignorance accumulated over ages gets cleared with education. When the darkness of ignorance is lifted, the light of joy of the Sun, dawns. This is what has been referred to here by Kumaraguru. Such an education gives us four types of advantages.
They are morality, material things, pleasure and liberation. It is only through morality, material things, and pleasure that we can attain liberation. Instead of going through that route, if we master

education then it is possible to attain all the four things. This is what is said in the following song:

Aram porul inbam veedum payakkum
Purangkadai nallisaiyum koottum urunkaval onru
Utruzhiyum kai kodukkum kalviyin oongillai
Chitruyirukku utra tunai.

Similarly just as education brings laurels wherever you go, so also, if we worship the Goddess of learning Saraswati whole heart-edly, then alone she will bless us all with knowledge and wealth.

In the modern times, research is being conducted to a large extent both on the Earth and in the outer space. The foundation for all that is education alone. If that is not there, there will be no researches, no production, no growth of the economy of the country, and there will be no security as well, is it not?

For a man to live a worthy life, is education important or wealth? When we ask this question, the reply usually received is, what can be done with education Sir? If we have money, even a corpse will get up and salute!" pat comes the reply. However, money does not speak everywhere. If we do not have the wealth of knowledge, even the wealth that has been accumulated with enormous effort cannot be saved. Numerals and alphabets can be used only by those who have eyes, is it not? Those who do not have the wealth of numbers and writing are equal to the blind.

Importance of Education

An uneducated person may be a millionaire but if a message in English flashes on his mobile, we find him showing it to his neighbour asking him to read it out for him. Therefore, the importance of education does exist even today.

Just as education is important for a nation so also, it is essential for an individual, the house where he lives, and the society to which he belongs. Education does not merely benefit a single person. The society or community which is connected to him is also benefitted by it. The inventions of Engineers are used not by his family alone but the entire society. From the electric bulb invented by Edison to the Motor car by Henry Ford, the inventions have touched pinnacles of glory in their usage by the people of the world. The basis of this happiness is knowledge.

Whatever may be the occupation, the knowledge and the experience given by education should be willingly learnt by all of us.

Of late, the world over, we see innovative ways of thefts, bank robbery, tax evasion, eloping, cheating, murder, rape, sexual abuse, prostitution and such other activities have multiplied beyond limits. Are these people uneducated? No. Those who are engaged in these kinds of base and shameful activities include well educated and knowledgeable people.

The very purpose of education itself is to improve the culture of man. Simplicity, restraint, contentment with what one has, is what is needed. Why does the education induce people to engage in such debasing activities? The reason is that they got the formal education but they did not get the corresponding wisdom.

Education is like a sword. It could be used as a knife to kill or it could be used to conduct surgery and save someone's life as well. What is necessary is the wisdom to know for what purpose it is to be used. This being absent is the cause for such frauds, looting, murder etc. that have become rampant today.

The ability to get rid of this, and for blossoming of love and peace in our lives is inherent in worship of the Goddess of learning, Saraswati.

Animals and birds have been able to easily get their food and live their lives without any education. Therefore, we should not entertain the idea that we should get educated merely to earn a living for the sake of food alone. Education should make us useful and wealthy so that we may become ideal citizens for our own good and for the national benefit. This alone is the main goal of education.

Man should make use of his wisdom appropriately and with it work for the welfare of the world; his education should enable him to provide an understanding of his Creator, make him devoted to him. However much a person might have had bookish learning, if he forgets God, there will be no use of his learning.

It is only when man is aware that God is having a constant watch over his actions that he will hesitate to perform demeaning deeds. Some may argue that it is possible to control crime through law. If what they say was true then with the prevailing excellent legal framework and courts, how is it that murder, looting increasing on such a large scale?

The main reason is that man has lost the fear towards that Supreme that he will have to face punishment in the Kingdom of God for crimes done on the Earth. If education instills this realization in his mind and heart, then with growing age he will not get distracted towards the wrong paths. Even if he is persuaded he will not be interested in another man's belongings.

The knowledge that God is ever watchful, will imbibe the fear even while living, that he will have to face the consequences of his wrong deeds and the belief that he can enjoy the heavens for good actions done here will help in disciplining his life. Otherwise, he will go where his desires take him and there will be no limits to his lust. He will not only bring peril to himself, but the suffering and damage caused to others will have no limits due to his transgressions.

When we lead a life of sin and immorality quality, we become victims of people's curses, the curse of women, and the righteous people thereby making life on the Earth itself a hellish experience. They will accumulate sins which will haunt thme for another life time as well.

In the name of logic and analysis, it is ignorance to blast all beliefs. In the name of teaching justice, logical thinking objecting to the existence of God on the grounds of blind faith will not help in cultivating devotion among children. It will only encourage atheism and false beliefs.

Under the circumstances, is it not natural that the children growing in these conditions will be selfish and have a disregard for the well-being of others? Then murder, robbery, and cheating will spread its wings, and women will become victims to untold misery. Keeping this in mind, we should instill devotion to God in the minds of our children, and make them have a reverential fear of God and his powers. It would not be an exaggeration to say, that worship of Goddess Saraswati will beneficial.

At least once a year, worshipping the Goddess of learning, and singing her praise, will not only be a reaffirmation of the necessity of education but will also give it due importance and proper understanding.

What do you mean by understanding?

Education's use is to help in constructive ways. Instead of that if the education leads to the destruction of the people and the nation then such education is only an information bureau and nothing else. It is this kind of education that the western countries have received. That is the reason why they manufacture Atom bombs and threaten the security of other nations. Using terrorism they are sacrificing human lives and threatening developing nations with atom bombs. Burning up the world's resources is the result of wrong education alone.

But our culture and tradition is not so. The crime that cannot be corrected through law is rectified through the intelligent application of religious tenets and rituals. Therefore performing the Saraswati puja in a grand manner we can attain the wealth of education and maturity.

There are several secrets hidden in the form and appearance of Goddess Saraswati. Let us now look into them.

32

Secrets of the form of the Goddess

If one has a close look at the form of Goddess Saraswati then we will notice thatthere are several symbolic representations of learning.

There is a rivulet besides which Goddess Saraswati is seated on a rock holding the Veena in her hands. She is wearing a white sari and the area surrounding her is very calm and peaceful.

What does the picture depict? Life is like the rivulet that flows down from the mountain top. That which stabilizes our life is the rock like education. Otherwise, life will wash us away in her tide. The highest pinnacle of education is knowledge and wisdom which when obtained one will not be shaken by happiness or sorrow.

Goddess Saraswati is peacefully seated on a rock. Those who have arrived at the shores of knowledge have a depth like that of an ocean where there is stillness and peace.

The white silk sari that she wears is symbolic of sacredness and fame. White is purity, white is fame. Therefore education is a wealth that is worshipped sacredly by all and makes one world renowned.

She has a Veena on her lap and she is playing on it. Music endears all. There is no one who is not swayed by music. Not only man, even animals and birds are influenced by music.

When Krishna played on his flute, the cows and calves which were engrossed in grazing, stopped and got enchanted. In the enchanting sound of Krishna's flute, living beings forget themselves. Forgetting all enmity, forgetting all hunger, they get transported into the divine realm.

Periazhwar sings:

Chiruviralgal tadavi parimaara chengan koda cheyaavay
Koppalikka
Govindan kuzhal kondu oodinapodu
Paravayin ganangal vandu chuzhndu Padukadu kidappa
Paravayin ganangal kavizhndirangi kaalparappittu
cheviyaattakillave

The birds that have to fly up in the sky and circle around, forgetting their prey come to the Earth and lie on the ground as though someone has tied them down. They are so absorbed in the music that they have forgotten themselves and have also forgotten how to flap their wings. Similarly, the cows, forgetting to chew the grass that is in their mouths, are standing still lending all their ears to the music mesmerized by it.

When music is so enchanting to those with merely five sense organs, can human beings be left behind? Even dried up trees come to life like fresh leaves. That is why the embodiment of all arts, Goddess Saraswati is seen playing the Veena in her hands. The whole of creation comes under her spell.

That is not all. She is giving expression to a great secret by holding the book and the veena in her hands. However much one has learnt their learning is only a handful. That which is yet to be learned is enormous. A professor in a University who is a teacher to his students, is also a student to a number of other subjects which he has yet to learn and widen his horizons of learning.

Even though I am the goddess for learning, I am still learning; so also you too much live like that"; this is what is indicated subtly by the Goddess Mahasaraswati.

In the name of rational thinking, we are foolishly imbibing several blind beliefs and practices of the western countries and spending exorbitant sums of money.

I shall give you an example. How do we celebrate the birthday of a child? By blowing off the candle on the cake before cutting it, is it not? Is it auspicious to blow a lit flame or inauspicious? The Western countries do not have any idea about Shastras or traditions. They do not have them. But is the Indian culture like that?

Both blowing off the lit flame and cutting the cake in place of performing a homam for increasing the longevity are inauspicious. Adopting this and such practices is merely to impress the world that we are rational and modern and is only a waste of money. But the Saraswati Puja that our ancestors taught us was not like that. Is the expenditure on Saraswati puja a wasteful expenditure? Let us look into some of the arguments on the subject.

33

Is Saraswati Puja unnecessary?

The amazing qualities of the Goddess

She is mildness personified, has Sattwic qualities, on that score she is not to be taken lightly. If a Sadhu flares up, even a forest cannot contain him, is an old saying in Tamil which is applicable to her perfectly. If a person becomes arrogant that he has become highly educated, then she is quite capable of making him lick the dust.

Even Asuras like Chamban who had become powerful due to boons, were destroyed due to this pride of being highly learned.

Even when she holds a book in one hand, she can also be seen with the hammer, arrow, bell, chakra, plough, bow in some other instances as well. If one has to live successfully in this world, it is not sufficient to only be intelligent; but one should also be courageous; this is what she makes us understand.

The auspicious days for performing the Saraswati Puja are the Saptami, Ashtami and Navami, i.e. the 7th, 8th and 9th day after the New Moon.

As the Shakti of Brahma, having been born from the body of Brahma Himself, Goddess Saraswati is also known by the names of

Savitri, Gayatri, Brahmani. In the Saraswati Suktam of the Rig Veda she is addressed as Adhikarini.

Her pictures are used during the Tara worship. She is holding a book in her hand. It is indicative of worldly knowledge, practical experiences, consciousness, and the basic skills for development of trades.

The Akshara mala in her hands stands for meditation and the spiritual knowledge.

There is the sacred water in the pot on one hand representing production, sacredness and energy.

She plays the veena. It is the embodiment of music, a gallery of arts, indicative of compatability.

Vageeshwari, Chitreshwari, Tulja, Keertishwari, Antariksha Saraswati, Kata Saraswati, Neela Saraswati, Kini Saraswati, are the eight forms of Saraswati in which the Goddess is worshipped.

History speaks of Dandi Mahakavi having worshipped Kata Saraswati, King Shalivahan having worshipped Chitreshwari, and the Poet King Kalidas having worshipped her as Shyamala and having achieved great fame.

Method of Saraswati Puja

The place where the puja is to be performed should be cleaned with water. Rangoli is then drawn over the place. Wipe the photo of Goddess Saraswati clean with a cloth, and apply kumkum, sandalwood and put a garland of flowers on the photo.

In front of the Devi, on a plantain leaf, place flattened rice, puffed rice, raw sugar, and fruits. Place the required books next to it and sprinkle sandal wood paste and water and apply kumkum on top.

On another plantain leaf, place the offerings of cooked grams, sweet rice, tamarind rice, lemon rice etc.

Thereafter a garland made of red lotus, white lotus, roses and jasmine is put on the photo. Loose flowers are showered on top of the books.

White lotus is the favorite of Goddess Saraswati. She is the Goddess who wears a white sari and is seated on a white lotus.

Therefore performing her puja with white colored flowers like the white lotus, jasmine, is very beneficial.

Since Vinayaka is the first God to be worshipped in any puja it is customary to make a symbolic idol with Turmeric paste and place him in the puja. Chanting the sloka, *"Shuklam Bharataram Vishnum, Shashivarnam, Chaturbhujam, Prasanna Vadanam Dhyayet, Sarva Vighnopa Shantaye"* his puja is performed. This is then followed with the chanting of the 108 names of Saraswati and singing her praise with the Sakala Kalavalli sloka.

Among the slokas taught to children this is one of the first slokas after Shuklam Bharataram sloka.

Saraswati Namastubhyam Varade Kaamarupini
Vidhyarambham karishyami Siddhirbhavatu me sada.

It is a very simple sloka and easy to understand.

Saraswati – Devi Saraswati
Namastubhyam – our prostrations to you
Varade- one who grants boons
Kaamarupini- One who bestows all desires
Vidhyarambham-commencing of education
Karishyami- I begin
Siddhir bhavatu me sada- may all these be accomplished.

There is also the practice of installing a Kalash as prescribed and performing the puja as well. Installing the Kalash brings additional benefits.

It is auspicious to worship her on all the nine days of Navaratri. If that is not possible, performing the puja on the day of Saraswati puja along with family members will bring the blessings of all learning and the arts and the skills.

Some ask whether Saraswati Puja is necessary. Is it not an unnecessary expense? People even write and speak about it.

Is it correct to think in this manner?

We have made it customary to perform the Saraswati puja on that day at home and in the offices. There are even those who say that this puja is meaningless, is mere exhibitionism, wasteful expenditure and make fun of those who worship. Worship of the Goddess of learning and celebrating her is not a wasteful expenditure. Let such people think as they please. In that sense, everything can be a wasteful expenditure.

During marriage ceremonies, why is the need to prepare so many varieties of dishes? Purchasing and wearing such expensive clothes, are they really necessary? Why should women be dressed up so lavishly?

Wearing Gold and diamond jewellery is a waste, is it not? There are people who comment that a smile itself is an ornament for a woman." What needs to be done and the way it needs to be done, if done that way alone will bring out the inherent beauty.

I will not have wasteful expenditure at my wedding so I will wear only a half pant", -no bridegroom will say that. If he says so, nobody will accept him as a bridegroom in the first place. On the other hand he may be subject to ridicule and become a laughing stock.

Is it necessary to have a holiday for schools, colleges, offices, factories on the day of Saraswati Puja? Some ask, is it not the day when we have to read books?

In India it is the custom, tradition and practice that before the beginning of any auspicious work or activity, a puja is performed for its success and for removal of obstacles to its accomplishment. Accordingly, the goddess who has been the guiding force throughout our life by giving us the wealth of education, her worship is not misplaced in any way whatsoever and granting one day holiday for her worship is also not wrong. If that were not so, there won't be that enthusiasm among the students, teachers, or family members in performing the puja.

Even after the students have gone to school, why do we do puja? It is possible that the family members may be casual and assume that the children are studying, so why worry? Even if the puja is performed, there is no need for preparing the Naivedya, because there is no one to eat them will be their argument. Keeping all this in mind, our ancestors have made it customary for Saraswati Puja to be performed and to have a holiday on that day. At least on that one day, we should devote our time and energy to worship and sing the praise of the Goddess of learning and arts, Saraswati Devi.

Even though there is so much glory and importance in the worship of Goddess Saraswati, the fact that there are not many temples on this Earth devoted to her exclusively, is a matter of disappointment. What is the reason for this? Let us get to know this.

34

Why is there no temple for Goddess Saraswati?

As compared to other Gods, there are not many temples in India dedicated to the worship of Saraswati. What is the reason for this?

Brahmadev was engaged in the task of creation in his Brahma Loka. The Goddess of Arts played the Veena and was doing her duty by expressions of knowledge and speech through the people. Saturn's glance fell upon them which gave rise to the feeling of pride in both that each one was better than the other.

Brahma spoke highly of his own importance since he was engaged in the task of Creation of the world. Saraswati argued that it was she who was giving them the power of speech. As a result of the argument between them both cursed each other. Both of them were born on Earth in the Kingdom of Chola brahmin as a result as the son and daughter of a blind couple named Punyakeerti and Shobhana.

They, who were living peacefully in the Satya Loka, were born as brother and sister on the Earth and suffered here due to their own egoistic pride. This makes us understand that such fate not only befalls mankind but even the Gods have had to suffer because of their own bad karmas in an earlier birth.

If a person says that he is capable of doing a thing, then it shows his self-confidence. But when he starts speaking that it is possible only for him then it shows arrogance. This   arrogance is fated to bring down a person from the great heights to the depths below. This was demonstrated in the lives of Brahmadeva and Saraswati.

Both of them were born as children, suffered from diseases and pain, had to face hunger and poverty and came to live in destitution in the house of the blind couple. Both grew up into a marriageable age. The parents began their search for suitable bride and a bridegroom.

It was at that time that both of them were awakened to the Truth about themselves. They realized that they who were Brahma and Saraswati living as husband and wife happily in the Brahma Loka, were born here as brother and sister on the Earth. Now if they were to get married, the world would despise them. They would be humiliated.

A husband and wife should adjust with each other and work towards making the family a priority. If that does not happen, such kind of complications and sufferings will crop up. It was as if to demonstrate to the world that Mahashakti made this birth to happen was the conclusion drawn by both of them. With great mental agony they narrated what had happened to their parents.

With a view to have a solution they prayed intensely to Shiva to relieve them of this complicated and distressing situation.

Shiva manifested himself and said, "Since you both have been born as brother and sister in this lifetime, you both should not get married. Therefore, Saraswati Devi, should forget about marriage and continue to live on Earth as a Virgin and Brahma Deva, should return to Satya Loka and take care of the work of Creation" saying which he disappeared.

It is for this reason that Goddess Saraswati appears alone by herself even in the few temples where she has manifested and is seen without husband.

Where husband has no temple, I too shall not have one

Besides, there is another reason for this as well. She is Brahma Shakti, complete by herself. Therefore, she is the Goddess of arts, the source of knowledge of all arts. In spite of that she does not have any temples to her while all other Gods have temples dedicated to their worship. Where even under trees deities are installed and worshipped in every nook and corner, isn't it surprising that the Goddess of learning does not have that many temples dedicated for her worship?

Brahma has very few temples for him on the Earth like that at Pushkar and there is no regular pujas done for him as the other gods. He is not so popular. But is Saraswati so? She is celebrated the world over. Besides the Hindu religion, Buddhists and Jains too celebrate her. Even then, Goddess Saraswati does not have many temples in India.

It is customary for women to avoid getting popularity or fame when their husbands have been denied that or does not have that kind of privilege. They prefer living in their shadows and consider that itself as their decoration. When my husband does not have a temple, then why should I have one? I shall reside on his tongue, saying which Goddess Saraswati got herself installed on his tongue. This is the reason why she does not have a temple separately built for her.

In Kancheepuram, in the Kamakshi Amman temple, there is an altar for Saraswati Devi. But even there, she is not present as Saraswati, Brahma's wife, but as a Minister to Rajarajeshwari, by the name of Raja Shyamala Maha Saraswati. Even in the temples where Saraswati is sculpted on stone, those are not celebrated as the main deity with pujas etc.

She does not permit being celebrated when her husband has been denied such worship. That is why she does not have temples and daily worship by way of pujas there. However for those devoted to her and who desire to perform her puja she slightly slackens her strictness.

During the Navaratri festival she participates as one of the three main Goddesses and allows herself to be worshipped with puja. She does not expect separate temple or pooja for herself and remains aloof with detachment. This is wisdom. If we are to attain that wisdom, we have to worship her. If we attain the wisdom, there is no other thing that is required in this world. There will be no desire for anything. We can be immersed in nitya Ananda. It is the Goddess Saraswati who helps in the ripening of this wisdom.

Fools list

Education that imparts wisdom is useful for all times. If we have only informative knowledge there is a possibility of getting fooled. Let us look into a story related to this.

Some horse merchants approached the King of another country. They presented some high class breed among their horses to him. The King purchased them for a high price and enjoyed riding on them.

He immediately ordered for a thousand more from them.

They replied, that they were businessmen who bought and sold horses and so would like to have an advance amount for the required number of horses, from the King.

The King called out to his Minister and asked him to hand over a lakh of gold coins from the Treasury to the horse traders.

The Minister however, cautioned the King, saying that they were not traders from their own Kingdom. Therefore it would neither be advisable nor appropriate to hand over such a huge amount to them.

The King brushed it aside and said, "Am I a fool? Do as you are told."

Having no other choice, the Minister gave the one lakh gold coins to the traders and saw them off. A month passed by and still there was no sign of the horses.

One night, when the King was in an intoxicated condition, he called his Minister and asked him to prepare a list of all the fools in his Kingdom.

Accordingly the Minister prepared a list and handed it over to the King the next day.

The first name on that list was that of the King. The King's fury on seeing this was beyond limits. He asked the Minister, "What is this! Why is my name on top of the list of fools?" he screamed.

"O King! Not knowing the past records of the businessman who came from other countries, and without any reference or credentials, you gave one lakh gold coins to them. Isn't it a foolish thing to do? That is the reason why I put your name on top of the list." The Minister replied calmly and obediently.

"What will you do if they bring the horses?" the King asked angrily.

"I shall remove your name and write theirs" replied the Minister teasingly.

If we do not have the wisdom to think in a balanced way, we will have to face heavy losses in our life, is the moral of the story.

The wisdom to think constructively and fairly that will help us in handling life's challenging and sorrowful situations is through education. Goddess Saraswati is the Goddess of all arts and learning. If we surrender at her feet, we shall be free of short comings and can lead a peaceful life.

There have been many who have attained great status and positions in life by worshipping Saraswati Devi. Among those are Pundits, great poets, and literary scholars, some of whom we shall acquaint ourselves with, in the next chapter.

35

The Goddess that altered
the course of the river

There are several instances in the literary works highlighting the fact that all success and prosperity are showered on those who bow down to Goddess Arulvani (Saraswati).

Two literary giants, who were called the Ilansuryan and Mudusuryan, got together on the banks of the river Pennaiattru in the Shiva Kshetra of Tiruvamattur, and sang. In this theyhad mentioned that the temple is located on the western banks of the river.

In fact, it is on the eastern banks of the river that the temple is located. During the inaugural presentation of the Sthalapuran, those who were in the know of the location questioned them as to how you sing that the temple is on the western banks while it is on the eastern banks, is it a mistake? They expressed their disagreement.

"Goddess Saraswati lives on our tongues. Her words are what we write. Therefore we are not responsible for what we sing, Kalaimagal does not lie" they argued.

That night a miracle happened. It rained heavily. Due to the intensity of the rains, the River changed its course and started flowing in a different direction. Now the temple is in the western banks. Considering the dilemma of the scholars, in one night, the one who could have changed the course of the river is only the gracious Mother Kalaivani, Goddess Saraswati is what is revealed by this incident.

Mother who raised the platform

The notable quotation of Poet Kalamegam is that we shall attain all that we need by bowing to Naamagal(Goddess Saraswati), the goddess of arts.

Kalamegam was one poet from whom poetry flowed like a perennial river due to the blessings of Kalaivani. Once, listening to others, the King of Tirumalai, instead of honoring him like the other scholars insulted him. Instead of reserving a seat for him, he made him to sit on the floor with others, with the intention of humiliating him.

But will Kalaimagal, allow her son to be insulted in a congregation of scholars? Certainly not! isn't it?

Understanding that the King is insulting him, poet Kalameg prayed to Kalaivani:

Vellaikkalai udutti Vellai Panipoondu
Vellai kamalatte Veetriruppal – Vellai Ari Asanattil Arasarodu
Yennai sariyasanamvaitta Thai.

Immediately, the throne on which the King was seated grew a little in height on one side. Kalameg went next to the King and sat down comfortably. The people and the King when they saw this realized their mistake and honored the great poet who was truly blessed by the Goddess Kalaivani.

Undisturbed sleep

Goddess Saraswati who was humble before her husband, on several occasions has risen to save humanity along with Brahma. We can see one such incident in the Ramayana.

Kumbakarna started intense Tapas to Brahmadeva lasting for a thousand years. His demand was immortality. If that was fulfilled, the Asura would live forever and be a source of perpetual harassment of the Devas. Brahma was worried because of this demand from him.

To end Brahma's distress, Saraswati, the Saras Vaani, the goddess of all arts, came to his rescue. Brahmadeva appeared before Kumbakarna who was doing intense penance to destroy all the Devas. At the same time, Goddess Kalaivani took her seat on his tongue. Not knowing this, Kumbakarna, bowed down to Brahma, and "I want one boon" he said humbly.

"What boon do you want" asked Brahma with a smile.

Kumbakarna said, "I want endless Nidra"

The misplacement of one letter completely changed the boon that he asked for. What he desired was "endless Nitya" or life without death but what was spoken by his tongue was "endless Nidra" that is continuous sleep. This drama was staged by the Gods written by Goddess Saraswati, using Kumbakarna as the actor for guarding that which was exclusive to the Gods.

Due to the boon of Nidra he became Kumbakarna. The Gods' fears were vanquished. He started spending his life eating and sleeping in the palace of Ravan.

Besides the Devas, Kalaivani, pleased with her devotees, namely the poets, authors of literary works and scholars, have always protected them from difficulties and testing times. We can find such instances in the lives of intellectuals and great men to a large extent. History has recorded them.

Some such instances have occurred in the life of the great scholar Kambar thereby showing her benevolence on him and her expression of her love for him.

36

Kambar and Kalaivani

The daughter of the Emperor of the Chola Kings, Amravati and Ambika pati, the son of Kambar fell in love with each other. This was admonished by Ottakuthar. He informed the King and tried to create bad blood between the King and Kambar. He wanted to use the occasion to somehow take his revenge on Kambar.

One day he arranged to invite Kambar and Ambika pati to lunch at the palace. This was a trick to catch the lovers red-handed. Not knowing this, Kambar and Ambika pati arrived at the palace.

Arriving at the palace, Ambika pati began getting amorous feelings like the horripilations of a lion. He happened to glance at his beloved damsel in the corridors of the palace. He became excited.

He forgot himself. The next moment he started singing soulfully thinking of Amravati, "*Itta Adi nog yedutta Adi Koppalikka Vattil sumandu Marungasaya*"

Finding the situation getting out of hand, Kambar interrupted.

"*Kotti kizhango kizhangendru kooruvaal Naavin Vazhangosai Vaiyam Perum*" he completed the song.

The whole song goes like this:

"*Itta Adi noya yedutta Adi Koppalikka Vattil sumandu Marungasaya*

Kotti kizhango kizhangendru kooruvaal Naavin Vazhangosai Vaiyam Perum"

The King noticed this. Ottakuthar, "O King! Did you notice him? See how he sang the love song to the beloved in his heart with his intention set on our Amravati? If Ambikapathy, son of Kambar who composes for kavi for fives and tens starts loving the King's daughter, what will the world think? He should be immediately punished and put behind bars" shouted angrily.

The King shook his head in agreement. He called out to the security guard close by.

Immediately Kambar interfered and said, "O King! I beg you not to be in haste! Please do listen to what I too have to say."

"It is true that my son sang a song with a girl in mind. But it was not your daughter. In the hot Sun, with the basket on her head, his feet walking on the parched hot mud path, unable to walk due to pain, a girl was selling some roots in the street. It was with her in mind that he sang that song."

The King sent the security guard and ordered him to go and see if there was any such girl in the street and if so, to bring her in.

The guard went outside and found an old woman selling some roots in a basket and brought her in.

Seeing this, Koothar was shocked. Kambar bowed down.

Koothar was annoyed that his dream was spoilt. The King was convinced that what Kambar said was the truth.

The woman who came there was Mother Kalaivani.

In this manner, the goddess manifested for the sake of her devotee, Kambar in the heat of summer, as an old woman with a basket on the head selling roots.

This is the classic example of the love that she showers on her devotees.

I am a slave to Ponni

Let us look at a story of Kambar attributed to Karna Parampara.

Jealous over Kambar's fame and the consequent anger, once, Ponni, a danseuse in the King's palace was sent to Kambar and she was asked to get in writing on a palm leaf from him, "I am Dasi Ponni's slave."

Initially she refused, but bribing her with a hundred gold coins, she was persuaded to change her mind; she became bold enough to humiliate Kambar.

One she met Kambar in an isolated place. Through her songs and dance she infatuated him. He too got fascinated by her artistic skills.

Having waited for this opportunity, the Dasi said, "Sir, for maidens like me, being praised in this way can be the result of meritorious deeds over several life times."

Kambar said, "I have truly become a slave to your exquisite singing and dance."

"If that is so, will you write on a palm leaf, that I am a slave of Dasi Ponni" and give it to me?" begged Ponni.

The infatuated poet, whose mind was lost in the attention of the young lady, immediately picked up a writing pen and wrote on a palm leaf and gave it to her.

Ponni brought it and gave it to the scholars. They were more than satisfied. She went home happily.

Armed with the palm leaf, those jealous scholars went to the King and showing it to him questioned the King on Kambar's character. They said, "See what kind of a poet is he! He has stooped down to the level of a Dasi and become a slave to her. See what he has written on a palm leaf." They said making fun of the poet.

The King was furious. He immediately ordered that Kambar be brought before him.

When he arrived, he showed him the palm leaf and asked, "Was this written by you?" His eyes darted like flames of fire.

Taking the palm leaf in his hand, Kambar looked at it. "Yes, I had written it" he said calmly.

"Don't you feel ashamed for writing like this?"

The scholars looked at each other and exchanged knowing smiles.

"What is there to be ashamed in that? Every word written on it is true."

"Chi... Chi... A poet who is loved and respected by a Chola King and the people of his kingdom is writing that he is a slave to a danseuse who dances shamelessly in public! You have put a Chola King to shame!" screamed the King.

"O King! You seem to have misunderstood what I said," replied Kambar slowly.

Hearing this, not only the King but even the name slayers were shocked.

"What1 Have I misunderstood?"

"Yes! Undoubtedly!"

"You have written that you, Kamban is a slave to Dasi Ponni. This is clear is it not? How can it be misunderstood?" asked the King.

"O King, in that sentence the letter Da means Thai, mother. And si means Shri which stands for auspiciousness. Ponni means golden, and stands for the golden colored Mahalakshmi to whom I am slave. I, Kamban is slave to Mother Mahalakshmi" is what I have written."

Attributing any other meaning to this will not be correct. I have written it with this meaning in mind" Kambar concluded.

Hearing this King was happy. The jealous pundits dropped their heads. It is this Goddess Saraswati, who had blessed him with the power of speech that Kambar worshipped in his heart.

The Goddess who gave her anklets

Kambar has composed a song in praise of Goddess Saraswati called Saraswati Andadi. This is the drama created by Kalaivani for the composition of that song. Let us get to know that story.

Kamban, who was known to be a great scholar and poet had great devotion to Kalaivani. When he faced difficult times, Kalaivani would console him saying, "Son, do not worry". Stories of her being by his side and having saved him have been narrated. Kalaivani incarnated as an old lady selling roots in order to save him which we saw earlier.

In order to save him from humiliation, there is the incident of she having bestowed her grace by removing the anklets from her feet and handing them over to him.

Due to the humiliation faced by him at the hands of the Chola King, Kamban left that Kingdom and arriving at the palace of Chera King served him without disclosing his identity. He would fold the betel leaves beautifully and give the King and engage him in delightful talks on literary matters.

Coming to know of the closeness between Kamban and the King, the other Pundits and dignitaries in the King's court started despising this. They plotted to somehow bring a controversy and get Kamban insulted and removed from the palace.

They brought a barber and arranged for him to meet Kambar and get him to say that Kambar was his brother. When Kambar came to know of this he felt sad. One could go to Rameshwaram but Saneeshwaran would still get there: he thought to himself; as if to confirm that; even though he had left Chola Kingdom in disgust, the troubles from jealous enemies doesn't seem to stop.

He prayed to Saraswati Devi. She said, "Kamban, do not worry. I am giving you one of my anklets. Make use of this and foil their plot to cheat you."

The next day, when Kambar went to the palace, he handed over the single anklet to the King and said that this was his tribute.

The brightness of the anklet, and its divine glow, fascinated the King tremendously. In my life time I have seen several kinds of gemstones and jewellery, but I have not seen one as beautiful and exquisite as this one, he said. Kambar, you have me only one anklet, where is the other one? He asked.

When I and my brother divided the anklets between us, this is the one I got as my share. The other one is with my brother he said.

Immediately, the King sent forth his guards to bring the other anklet from the barber.

When they went to the barber, he said, that he did not have any anklet.

When they found him refusing to accede to their polite request, they decided to tie him and beat him up with a stick. The Senapati tied him up and started beating with a whip.

The barber screamed. He said, "O Sir! I shall tell you the truth. Kambar is not my brother. Your royal Pundits threatened me and asked me to say so. I have not committed anything wrong. Sir, Senapati please forgive me. Please leave me. Tell them not to kill me" he pleaded to them with folded hands.

It was then that the King came to know of the truth. The person who was serving him all these days was one of the stalwarts among poets, Kambar. He was overjoyed.

He looked at him and asked, "Whose anklet is this? How did you get it?"

"O King! This is the anklet of the Goddess whom I worship and pray to daily, Kalaivani." Saying this, Kambar sang in praise of the Goddess, the composition which came to be celebrated as "Saraswati Andadi".

Aayakalaigal Arupattinaangkinayum
Eya unavirkkum Ennammai – Tuya
Uruppalingu Polvaal em ullathin ulle
Iruppal Ingu Vaaraadu Idar.
Padiga Niramum Pavala Chevvayum
Kadikamazh Puntamaraipol kaiyyum – Tudiyidayum
Allum Pagalum Auavratamum Tudhittal
Kallum Chollaado Kavi.

He started showering praise on Goddess Saraswati. Let us look at another song written by him.

Oruttiyai Onrumilla En manattil Vandu Tannai
Iruttiya Venkamalattiruppalai Ennen kalaitoy
Karuttiyai Imbulanum Kalangaamal Karuttai Yellam
Tiruttiyai yaanmaraven Disainaanmugan Deviyaiye.

The one who picked my mind which who had no good intentions at all, she who is seated on a white lotus, one who has the mind soaked in the sixty four arts, whose has made all her sense her servants and not allowing it to run randomly, having controlled them, she the wife of the four-faced one, Brahmadeva, She is the Devi whom I cannot forget. This is the essence of the song.

There are in all about 30 songs sung in praise of the Goddess Kalaivani in Kambar's book of compositions.

Those who chant the Saraswati Andadi on the day of Saraswati puja will be blessed with all kinds of benevolence.

Listening to these songs, Kalaivani was so pleased that she danced to the sounds from the one anklet on her leg and celebrated his compositions. Later, she gave him her darshan and asked for her other anklet back.

No sooner than he handed over the anklet that was given to the King, it instantly disappeared. For some time, the feet of Kalaivani which had worn the two anklets appeared like a flash of lightening and then vanished.

Those who were witness to this miracle were so astonished that some of them fainted, some felt horripilations all over the body, and still others who out of jealousy had tried to harm Kambar, now fell at his feet and asked them to be forgiven.

Thus, Kalaivani has always stood by her devotees and this is one story where she had given her own anklet that she wore on her feet and also gave her darshan to the people.

37

Saraswati Devi worshipped by Kambar

Mannavanum Neeyo Valanadum Unado
Unnai Arindo Tamizhai Odhinen – Ennai
Viraindetru Kollada Vendundo, Undo?
Kurangetru Kollada Kombu.

Are you the only King in the whole world? Chera, Pandyas are also there. Is the Chola, the only Kingdom where I can live? Certainly not! There are several other prosperous countries where I can live. Have I learnt Tamil depending on you alone?

Will another branch of a tree refuse to accept a monkey that has jumped from one branch of the tree? Similarly, if I leave your country and go to any other country, the King of that land will immediately welcome me and accept me. Singing the above song with this meaning, Kambar angrily left Chola country.

A few years before his death, Kambar had handed over the idol of Saraswati Devi that he had been worshipping with puja to one of the Chera Kings. He had requested that puja was to be performed on every day of the nine days of Navaratri to the idol. Accepting to the request, the King performed its puja accordingly. As per that tradition and practice, even today the idol is seated on an elephant and brought in a procession with all pomp and splendor to the Padmanabha swami temple at Tiruvananthapuram during the Navaratri festival and its puja performed in a grand manner.

Kambar's idol of Kali which he worshipped is about 2000 years old. Beneath her feet there is an etching of the form of a scholar which is believed to be Kambar according to the archaeological researchers. Beneath the Goddess's left leg there an idol which appears to be a dancing Nandi.

When the goddess had danced in anger, the whole creation of animate and inanimate objects also danced with her. The Trinity of Devas, all the species of animals, the plants, and the trees too moved from their places and danced. They trembled in fear. They wondered in fear and confusion as to how her dancing could be stopped.

Nandi got an idea. He went before the Mother and he too danced. Seeing him dance, Kali Devi started to laugh. Her anger subsides. She gets Nandi Deva to become quiet and settle down near her feet according to the reports from ancient times.

Let us get to know this a little more in detail.

When Kambar lost his beloved son Ambika Pati he was grief stricken and left the Chola country. He walked on foot and arrived at the Chera Kingdom. He meets the King and hands over the idol of Mother Saraswati, he had worshipped and performed puja whcih for all these years, and requesting him to take care of it and perform its puja. He passes away after a few days.

The King promised that every Navaratri he would perform the Saraswati Puja to the idol and have celebrations for her. However it was not easy to perform the puja for the Devi and conduct the festivities. The King Martanda who succeeded him to the throne was faced with several challenges and problems.

He however slowly and steadily gained victory over them. Several Kings from other countries tried dethrone him and seize to the Kingdom. But the King faced them all bravely and turned victorious. He completely eliminated them and ensured that his entire lineage would not suffer from their invasions.

He firmly believed that Mahasaraswati Devi's blessings and grace alone ensured his protection. All those who followed him in the lineage showed keen interest in some form of Fine arts or the other like music, painting etc. They were particularly devoted to music and promoted it to a great extent.

It was in the same lineage that saw the rise of Swati Tirunal Maharaja. Tirunal Maharaja ruled nearly 300 years ago. He shifted his capital from Padmanabhapuram to Tiruvananthapuram. But the idol of Saraswati Devi worshipped by the Kings over the years was left back at the palace. Every year she was taken for the Navaratri puja with all honors on a decorated elephant to the puja Mandap specially set up at the Anantapadmanabha Swami temple at Tiruvananthapuram. The procession of the Goddess seated on an Ambari on the elephant is glorified by devotees all along the way.

Do you know what the uniqueness in this is? In every temple it is only the Utsava idol that is taken outside the temple in procession. But here, instead of the Utsava idol, the idol of Saraswati Devi given by Kambar long years back is taken in procession. The Kings and all the successors in the family, honoring the word of promise given to Kambar continue the tradition to this day.

Before the idol of the Devi is taken out for the procession, a lamp is lit and kept in the place of the idol. The Devi's idol remains at Padmanabhapuram for all the nine days during which period when the idol is not there here, puja is performed to the lamp as representing the Saraswati Devi.

The first deity to be worshipped at the Tiruvananthapuram Navaratri Festival is Mother Mahasaraswati Devi. During the first three days she is worshipped as Mahasaraswati Devi, the next three days, she is worshipped as Mahalakshmi and the last three days she is worshipped as Mahakali.

At one point of time, chanting of the Vedas, Granth Puja, Ayudha puja, discourses from the Puranas, musical concerts and other such programs were organized during the Festival. Presently that glory is enjoyed by musical concerts which are given greater preference.

The reason for this is King Swati Tirunal. He had composed nine Kirtanais in Rag Shankarabharanam, Kalyani, Shuddha Saveri,

Kaveri, Todi, Bhairavi, Bandhuvarali, Naatta Kurunji, and Arabi in praise of Mother Saraswati. These are sung at the Mandap during the Navaratri festival.

Every day during the Navaratri festival celebrations, a specific Keertana based on a particular Rag is sung in a concert commencing at exactly 6 in the evening and concluding at 8:30 pm. No one is allowed to sing even a minute beyond 8:30 as per the instruction of the King. Besides, no one is also allowed to clap hands in appreciation of the musical concert as this concert is dedicated to the worship and remembrance of Goddess Saraswati Devi in the form of a musical offering.

The Navaratri Mandap is made out of wood. There are lamps lit on all four sides of the Mandap. Foreigners and people of other religions are not allowed into the Mandap. Only male singers are allowed to sing in the Mandap. The women are not permitted. Besides, there are separate arrangements for members of the royal family, both men and women, to listen to the concert. Others can enjoy the concert seated outside.

Electrical equipments are not used for the occasion. Inverted mud pots are piled around the Mandap. This helps in maintaining the volume of sound and the broadcast can be multiplied several times over. In other words it is the equivalent of the loudspeaker of the modern times.

These mud pots are of different sizes. Their mouth pieces are also of different sizes. This is why the sound echoes from all sides. These pots are tied together from several angles.

The celebrations to Saraswati Devi as per Kambar's instructions have been going on for over a thousand years which itself is a surprising thing.

Next to Kambar, the one who has been on the receiving side of the benevolence and blessings of Kalaivani is Shri Kumara Gurubar Swami. He had learnt the Hindustani language in one night and had discussions with the Badshah the next day. How Saraswati Devi blessed and influenced his life is the subject matter of our next chapter.

38

Meenakshi's gift to Kumara Gurubar

Having nine Kailash Kshetras on her banks and nine Tirupatis set up, the Tamirabharani River is truly magnificent. The Tirupati named Shri Vaikunth to the north of the river has a town named Kailash situated close by. A poet by the name of Shanmuga sigamani and his wife Shivakama Sundari lived in that town, like one soul in two bodies. They were born in a family of Shivite and were greatly devoted to Muruga.

They had a male child. While they felt very blessed, they were at the same time worried as well. The reason being, the child did not speak a single word till the age of five.

They prayed intensely to Lord Muruga, "You alone are our savior. Therefore it is your responsibility to make our son address us as Mother and father." They fasted, undertook vows, and performed pujas, but to no avail.

Broken hearted with grief, they took the child and went to the Muruga temple at Tiruchendur. They decided to stay there and prayed to Muruga to bless the child with the capacity of speaking.

One day, Senthil Muruga blessed the child; the child called "Amma" and calling out "Appa" he went and wrapped his hands around his father's neck. What could be more joy giving to them?

They felt extremely grateful to the Senthil Murugan who had blessed their son with speech. With tears in eyes they fell at his feet and took leave of him.

That miraculous child was Kumara Gurupar. He authored a book titled "Kandar Kalivenba" singing the praise of Lord Muruga who blessed him with the Siddhi of speech. Later he wrote an essay on the Lord of Kailash who manifested in their town, under the title of "KailaiKalambakam".

His devotion and detachment increased. He started a pilgrimage to each of the Shiva Kshetras; he prayed and sang in praise of the Lord and compiled a compendium of Tamil songs. Coming to Madurai he spent some time there.

At that time, he composed a collection of songs called Madurai Meenakshi Amman Pillai Tamil and this was introduced by King Tirumala Nayagar at his palace. The songs got everyone's appreciation.

No doubt everyone present was moved. But a seven year old little girl wearing green silk dress and garland of beads walked in amidst the crowd and came forward and sat on the lap of Kumara Guruvar. At the time of inauguration of the "PillaiTamil" the child took off the garland of beads from her neck and put it around the neck of Kumara Gurupar and disappeared.

That little girl was none other than the Goddess of the temple at Madurai, Meenakshi Amman. On knowing which, all present there were spell bound. It was as though Madurai Meenakshi herself had come there in the form of the little girl, listened and enjoyed the songs of Kumara Guruparar and as though by way of felicitation she presented the garland of beads thereby enhancing the prestige and uniqueness of the book.

Seeing this, the King of Tirumalai Nayagar also honored him in various ways and felicitated him.

Kalaivani teaches another language

Kumara Gurupar's urge to be initiated into Saivite philosophy- Shiva worship and code of conduct and become a Sanyasi began to gather increasing sense of urgency as days passed by for which he started looking out for a suitable guru. At that time under the tutelage of Dharmapuram Mutt in the Thiru Kailasha tradition, appointed as the fourth successor, Shri Masilamani Desikar was well versed in Saivite philosophy. Kumara Gurupar approached him and humbly asked him to be initiated by a deeksha into Saivite philosophy and code of conduct.

As per the traditions of the Mutt, if a person is to be given Deeksha and to be initiated into Sanyas, he has to have gone on pilgrimage to several Shiva Kshetras and had the darshan Shiva. More specifically, he should have visited Kashi and only after his return from there he would be initiated into Sanyas. Guruparar was informed accordingly.

"Swami, it will take several months to go to Kashi and return; will this body last that long? Is it possible? Can you please tell me any other way out?" asked Kumara Guruparar.

Seeing the maturity of the student and his determination the Guru was very pleased. Still, in order that rules are not transgressed and if it was not possible to go to Kailash, he should spend some time at Chidambaram was the condition that he put on Kumara Guruvar.

Kumara Guruparar left for Chidambaram. On the way he halted and prayed at the Vaitheeswaran temple. In praise of the Lord Kumara Guruswamy, he composed one Pillai Tamil. Later he went to Chidambaram and after having the darshan of Lord Nataraja; he stayed there for a while and wrote a Prabandham titled Chidambara Mummanikkovai.

After some years, he met his spiritual guru at the Mutt and asked him to give him the ochre robes. Realizing that the student was ready, he gave deeksha to Kumara Guruparar. As an expression of his love and devotion and as a mark of his respect for his guru who had initiated him into Sanyas, Kumara Guruparar wrote an extraordinary Prabandham titled Pandara Mummanikkovai, thereby marking an expression of his gratitude to him as well.

Later, he travelled to several other places and had the darshan of the Lord. Taking leave of his Guru, he went to Delhi and met the Badshah there. He had no knowledge of Hindustani language while the Badshah on the other hand did not know Tamil language. So, in order to be able to converse with him effectively, he decided that he had to learn the Hindustani language.

He prayed to Kalaivani and wrote a book of songs in praise of the goddess of all arts and asked that he be given the knowledge of that language. In a single night he attained the Siddhi of the knowledge of the Hindustani language. Kalaivani blessed him with the knowledge and a great understanding of the Hindustani language.

He then had a whole hearted dialogue with the Badshah. Seeing the knowledge of Kumara Guruparar in Hindustani language, his humility, his restraint, and above all his devotion, the Badshah was very impressed and honored him greatly. The Badshah was awed and inspired on learning that his knowledge of the language was due to Kalaivani's blessings and grace.

He offered him a permanent place of residence on the banks of the river Ganges at Kashi near Kedar ghat. Kumara Guruparar established an ashram there and began his spiritual work there. He started discourses in Tamil and Hindustani on Kambar Ramayana. It used to be attended by Tulsidas.

In the later period, when Tulsidas wrote the Ram Charita Manas in Hindi language he included there in some of the views of Kamba Ramayana and thereby enhanced the prestige of Tamil language as well.

In this manner Kumara Guruparar carried on his activities for several years at his ashram and once came to Dharmapuri to meet his spiritual guru. He then returned to Kashi and resumed his work. After some years, on the third day after the Full Moon in the month of Vaikasi he attained salvation at the feet of Lord Shiva.

By the benevolence and Grace of Saraswati he wrote several books and plays. If the students read the Sakalakalavalli Malai written by him with devotion, their memory will improve. The language skills will increase. Their ability to understand will become better. They will get better marks and thereby will be able to secure better opportunities for higher education.

Hence, the Sakalakalavalli songs are given below with meanings in a simple language. Read it with understanding and secure merits in your education.

39

Sakalakalavalli garland of songs

Ventamaraikkandri Ninpadam taanga En Vellaiyulla
Tandaamaraikkum Tagadu Kolo Sakamezhum Alittu
Undaan Uranga Ozhittan Pittaga undaakkum Vannam
Kandaan chuvaikol karumbe sakala Kalaavalliye   *1*

During the time of the great annihilation of the seven worlds, Mahavishnu absorbs them all into his stomach and rests as a small child on the leaf of a banyan tree floating on the waters of the ocean. Rudra who destroys everything dances his Tandava of death like a man out of his senses. Brahma who is the Creator of the Universe is enjoying you like a sugar cane stick. Don't you love sitting on a white lotus? My heart too is white and pure free of any cunningness. Will your feet not touch there too? Give me that good fortune.

Naadum Porutchuvai chorchuvai thoytara Naarkaviyum
Padumpaniyil Panittarulvaai Pangaya Aasanattil
Kudum Pashupor kodiye Kanatanakkundrum Aimpaal
Kaadum chumakkum Karumbe Sakala Kalaavalliye   *2*

O One who is like the beautiful creeper made of pure gold! Beautiful breasts, thick long and black hair like a dense forest! Bless me with the skills of endearing speech and tasteful interests, so that my work of composing songs is appreciated and preferred by all in this world.

Allikkum chezhuntamizh Tellamudu Aarndu Un Arutkadalil
Kullikkumpadi Endru Kudum Kolo Ulangkondu Telli
Telikkkum Panuval Pulavor Kavimazhai chindakandu
Kalikkkum kalapa Mayile Sakala Kalaavalliye   *3*

Just as a peacock dances when the darkening clouds appears, Kalaivani, you who sways like the peacock rejoice listening to the deep and meaningful wisdom of gifted poets, when will the day arrive when we will be able to enjoy your pure Tamil amrutham and be drowned in your ocean of grace?

Tukkum Panuval Turaitoynda kalviyum Chorchuvai Toi
Vaakkum Peruga Panittarulvai Vadanur Kadalum
Tekkum Chezhuntamizh Chelvam Um Tondar Chennavinindru
Kaakkum Karunaikkadale Sakala Kalaavalliye   *4*

Kalavalli, I pray that you bestow upon me the ability to learn the most popular songs, deeply contemplative literature, the literary works in Sanskrit, and the ocean of writings in Tamil and gather the wisdom and pleasure from all of them.

Panjapi Idantaru Cheyyapporpaadapam Kerukam En
Nenjattadattu Alaraadadenne? Nedundaat kamala
Tanjattu Vasam Uyartton Chennavum Agamum Vellai
Kanjat Tavisu Ottirundaai Sakala Kalaavalliye   *5*

O Kalaavalli, you who are seated on the white lotus and in the heart and tongue of Brahmadeva, Your soft cotton like lotus feet are for some reason refusing to be seated in the ocean of my heart; please me with that grace O Kalaavalli!

Pannum Bharatamum Kalviyum Teenjol Phanuvalum Yaan
Yennum pozhudu yelidu Eida Nalkaai Ezhuda Marayum
Vinnum Puviyum Punalum Kanalum Vengalum Anbar
Kannum Karuttum Niraindai Sakala kalavalliye   6

O Goddess! You who are encompassing the Vedas which no one has ever written and the five elements such as land, water, fire, air and space, please bless me with the ability of creating music and songs and sweet sounding words filled literature that capture the hearts of people who listen to it. Please be merciful.

Paattum Porulum Porulal Porundu Payanum Enbal
Kuttumpadi Nin kadaikkan Nalkai Ulam Kondu Tondar
Theettum Kalaittamizh Teembal Amudam Telikkum Vannam
Kaattum Velodimappede Sakala Kalavalliye   7

Please fill me with the ability to compose songs that are good, filled with messages for an ideal living, and which are beneficial to those who listen or read them. Just like the ability of the Swan to sift through a mixture of milk and water and drink only the milk, may my songs be such as to enable sifting through and picking up of the sublime thought that are elevating O Sakala Kalavalli, bless me with your benevolent gaze.

Cholvirpanamum Avadaanamum kavi Sollavalla
Nalviddhaiyum Tandu Adimaikkolvai nalina Aasanam Ser
Selvikku Aridu endru Orukaalamum Chidayaamai Nalkum
Kalvipperum Selvappere Sakala Kalavalliye   8

Without giving room for me to lament that I did not have the blessings of Mahalakshmi seated on the lotus, O Sakala Kalavalli, bless me with the skills of oratory, ability to sing songs spontaneously, and creating literary works and compositions liked and appreciated by all and thereby making me indebted to You O goddess!

Sorkum Porutkum Uyiraam Meijnyanattin Totram Enna
Nirkindra Ninnai Ninaippavar Yaar? Nilamtoy Puzhaikkai
Karkum paadambuya Thaaye Sakala Kalavalliye   *9*

O Sakala Kallavalli! Your beautiful walk will put to shame the gait of an elephant or the graceful walk of a Royal Swan. You are the very embodiment of the sublime wisdom. You are always in my thoughts while I am standing, sitting, lying down or walking. O Goddess do not forget me!

Mankonda Venkudai Keezhaga Merpatta Mannarum En
Pankanda Alavil Paniyacheyvai!
Padaippon Mudalaam Vinkanda Deivam Palkodi Undenum
Vilambil Unpol
Kankanda Deivam Ulado! Sakala Kalavalliye!   *10*

There may be many gods who live in the universe starting from Brahma the God of Creation, but Sakala Kalavalli, there is no one else who manifests as the Goddess on merely our wishing.

The Kings who rule the Earth, even those who are the Emperors who rule over the Kings and even the Chakravartis, listen to my songs, O Sakala Kallavalli, make them gracious enough me to give me the deserving respect.

So far we have seen the glory of the Goddess of Knowledge, Saraswati and the incidents that portrayed her benevolent grace upon her devotees. Now let us see the places where she has manifested and the temples and places of worship dedicated to her.

40

Temples of Saraswati Devi

There is a temple of Saraswati Devi at Koothanur in Tamil Nadu. At the TillaiKali temple at Chidambaram there is an altar to Goddess Saraswati having the Veena in hand.

Koothanur Saraswati Devi

The Mahasaraswati Devi temple at Kuthanur is located in the Tiruvarur district, which is on the route from Mayiladunturai to Tiruvayur, near a village called Puntottam at a distance of about half a kilometer.

She is Ambika Mahasaraswati.

Site is Gnyana Peetham.

She is the Goddess of learning.

She has a rosary of beads or Akshara mala in her hand; she rides on a Swan and is showing the Chinmudra on her hand.

Mahasaraswati, the Goddess of Knowledge and arts is wearing a white silk sari; she is seated on a white lotus; she has an Akshara Mala in her upper right hand; she has the pot with the nectar of immortality on her upper left hand. Her eyes are brimming with mercy, and she has an eye on the forehead for bestowing knowledge.

Those who worship Saraswati Devi will be blessed with knowledge and wisdom. If you consider education as a means of gathering information then using it wisely to be of service to the country and the family becomes knowledge. Worship of the Goddess by students helps them to develop their capacity for higher education. When children are being first admitted to school, they are brought here to worship the goddess for receiving her blessings for success in their studies.

Praying to the Goddess regularly not only ensures proficiency in studies but also improves memory; it enhances the ability to exhibit that knowledge, improvise on the marks obtained, success at debating competitions and such other endeavors.

Abhirami Andadi says, "*Dhanam Tarum, Kalvi Tarum, oru naalum Talarvariya Manam Tarum*".

In the modern times, everyone is educated, some are highly educated, still they lament that they do not have the desired jobs. If this has to go away, then one should go to Kuthanur and worship Goddess Saraswati Devi soulfully.

When one prays to her, the Goddess of Knowledge will bless you with direction towards that education which will provide you with a job. This is what Abhirami Bhatt elaborates in his song by stating the objective first. By worshipping her, the students will be able to make use of the education acquired fruitfully and it will become a source of income for them; such education will become powerful.

Students, artists, writers, authors, painters, sculptors, artisans and craftsmen, handicrafts traders, all come to Koothanur and worship the Devi and pray for achieving success in their respective fields.

Ottakoothar

In order to be successful in the three main pillars of Tamil arts, namely, physics, music and dance, it is necessary to have the blessings of Goddess Saraswati. If one receives the benevolent grace of this Goddess, Ottakuthar says that of the sixty four arts, one can become proficient in sixty two of them. He was good at singing Bharani; he has sung Daksha Yaga Bharani, Muvarula; he was the Royal poet in the palace of the Chola Kings; his name is associated with the name of the town as well; due to the grace of Goddess Saraswati, he was the Scholar at the palace of the Cholas for three successive Kings. The respect accorded to him was equivalent to that of the King himself; in fact he was one step ahead of the King because of his erudition. People used to listen to him with all humility, bowing down with fingers over their mouth in respect and receive his instructions. Such was the dignity and honor with which he lived his life.

Normally, people only had fear toward the Kings who were very powerful. But with elders who had wisdom and knowledge as well, there is a respect along with fear, a kind of reverence. This is the beauty of education. Kalaivani gives that beauty to learning.

Some people will select a particular branch of education but will then get employed in a totally different field of activity and will be slogging there with disinterest and without any inspiration. Such people should go to Koothanur and pray to Goddess Saraswati to bring about a change. She blesses with change and happiness.

Saraswati's husband is the Creator Brahma. Saraswati is the essence of the Vedas essential for him to carry out the work of creation. She is the embodiment of Knowledge. Ordinary people like us, when we get two additional qualifications, think very highly of ourselves. But Kalaivani Devi Saraswati has the very manuals of Creation of this Universe, the Vedas themselves, and is showing the direction for her husband. But she has no pride or sense of superiority about it. She does not boast that this could happen only because of her. She is the brightness of knowledge like the Sun shining her light everywhere.

In spite of having so much glory, she is restrained, and has no pride or ego. She holds a bundle of palm leaves containing manuscripts, in one hand as though to demonstrate what we have learnt is very little and what is yet ot be learnt is very large. Our Goddess Saraswati truly embodies the statement of the Tirukkural which says, "*Paniyumaam Enrum perumai*" meaning The great are always humble.

If we humble down and surrender at her feet, our education will be useful for our whole life time. We will have a good livelihood. Our capacity for decision making will be good. It will yield good results. Above all it will bring peace.

Jnyanamum kalviyum nayamudan Kuda katra Viddhai narpalan
Nalki nanilatte Needuvazha Puntotta Arasalaaru Urai Jnyana Satyadi
Kuduveere.

Pulippani Siddhar sang what was stated above through this song.

A visit to Koothanur located on the banks of the river Arasu will bring all the blessings that Siddhar speaks about and the Goddess will definitely bless us.

Uniqueness of the Swan

We can see each of the Hindu Gods having a unique vehicle for themselves.

Saraswati Devi has the white Swan as her vehicle and she can be seen riding on it. White stands for superiority, fame, brightness, purity, and a freshness or newness.

The Swan has one quality which is not found in any other bird which has also been mentioned in the Itihasas and Puranas.

The Swan can separate milk and water from a mixture of milk and water and will drink only the milk. This has been mentioned in several places in our literature.

Those who worship Saraswati Devi, will get the wisdom to sift away that which is harmful and select only the good. This is the significance of the vehicle on which she rides.

What is held as knowledge today is a circle of light behind the head; this is not knowledge. Getting entangled in the bad influence of Maya, choosing to enjoy visual pleasures through eyes, and later realizing one's folly, regretting having let life go by uselessly, has become common among many these days.

Lack of knowing to select the right path, not knowing what is good for you, are the tortoises that are responsible for slowing down the pace of life. If you go to Koothanur and pray to Saraswati Devi, one's mind gets uncluttered and purified, confusions will vanish, decision making will improve thereby leading to success in life.

Students come to this temple and writing their desires on a piece of paper, they place it at the feet of Goddess Saraswati and leave after praying to her. They find this to help them by removing their inhibitions, bringing in them a renewed faith, and enabling them to face whatever the consequences fearlessly.

Separated lovers unite here

This place known as Arasalaaru is said to be holy and is said to unite lucky separated married couples. Once, an occasion arose when Gangadevi was required to be separated from Lord Shiva. She got separated from the matted hair of Shiva and started doing penance.

Lord Shiva got married to Parvati. Out of the flame from the third eye on the forehead, Karthikeya was created out of the flames. Karthikeya killed the Asura.

After killing Tarakasur, Gangadevi came running and embraced Lord Shiva. Mother Ganga who was separated came and embraced her husband Lord Shiva at this place Arasalaaru. It is in such a holy place that Saraswati Devi has manifested herself and is offering her blessings.

Mother Ganga manifested here in order to provide waters for the Abhishekha of Lord Shiva and she came to be known as Rudra Ganga and that is the Teerth here. It is filled with medicinal properties. Those who swim in her waters get cured of diseases.

It is said of this place that Bhogasiddar worship Goddess Saraswati here before proceeding to carve idols of Muruga of stone. All the thirty three crores of Gods, the King of Gods, Indra attribute their knowledge and take the darshan of this Goddess here for sustained and increasing wisdom. Brahma is present here along with Saraswati Devi as husband and wife and it is believed that taking their darshan at this temple will free us from rebirth.

How is that so? One may ask.

It is true that one gets cured of diseases. But of all diseases the most serious one is that of entanglement in the cycle of birth and death. In order to be free of this disease one requires Vairagya or detachment. One should have the dispassionate nature to be detached from the influence of Maya.

Knowledge is necessary for developing detachment. Saraswati Devi bestows this knowledge. Those who worship her not only get free from other kinds of diseases but also get rid of the disease of rebirth.

Mata Udal salitthal, Valvimaiye Kaal salithen
Vedavum kai salithu Vittane – Nadha
Iruppaiyur Vazhum shivane Matrumor Annai
Karuppayur Vaaramal Ka.

This song was sung by Pattinathar. Lamenting that the karmas done by us cause us to be born again and again, he says that having taken innumerable births, several mothers have carried us in their wombs and were fed up. Even we, after going through lifetimes after lifetimes, fed up with all the sorrows, lament, "Swami, enough of these sufferings".

All these pain; of taking repeated births that a person has to take that he should live his life in this manner; the one who writes all our destiny, that Brahma himself is said to have got fed up after writing thousands and thousands of such destinies of people. Therefore, going to the holy place of Iruppaiyur, Pattinathar is said to have prayed to Lord Shiva whose temple is there at this place, to not give him another birth and thereby giving him the punishment of having to give another mother the burden and pain of carrying him in her womb.

It is only when we get this knowledge that one will be free of desires in this world. Birth and death will stop. It is Devi Saraswati of Koothanur who gives us this knowledge and also shows us the way of getting rid of this disease of rebirth. The books on Saraswati Devi called Saraswati Andadi written by Kambar and also Sakala Kalavalli Mala of Kumara Guruparar have been composed and created for us.

One should go and have her darshan at least once. Along with education, you will also get the wisdom and prosperity in life. Koothanur is in Tiruvarur district. It is at a distance of half a kilometer from Poonthotam.

41

Other places of worship

We saw the existence of a separate temple for Saraswati Devi at Kuthanur in Tamil Nadu. Besides this, there is a temple separately for the Devi in Sringeri and Cuttack. Proper pujas are being performed for the Goddess at these temples.

In Andhra, there is a temple of Goddess Saraswati at a place called Basra.

In Kashmir on the Takt-e-Suleman hills there is a very ancient temple called Sarvagna Peetha.

In Tamil Nadu, at Kanyakumari, there is a temple of Saraswati Devi at Kulasekharapuram. The Devi in this temple is Ambika who was worshipped by Kavimani Desika Vinayakam Pillai.

Besides this, Saraswati Devi is worshipped at Tibet, Nepal, Indonesia and Japan. She is called Benzaiten.

Procedure for worship

Take a wooden board, wipe it clean and draw a Rangoli on it with white rice powder. Books are then piles upon it consisting of school text books, Ramayana, Mahabharata and other spiritual scriptures.

Elongated books, note books are placed at the bottom and the smaller books are placed above it in a neat pile in such a way that they look aesthetically beautiful and do not fall down. Books are the wealth of students. Therefore the sharp gaze of the Goddess Saraswati should fall on them. Therefore it is advisable to place a photo of Goddess Saraswati on top of the books.

Saraswati Devi is seated on a white lotus. She wears a white silk sari. Therefore we should offer her a garland of fragrant white flowers. She is the Guru of knowledge. The appropriate color for a Guru is yellow. Therefore her puja should be performed with yellow marigold flowers. Her archana done with white lotus flowers will bring added benefits. Performing her archana with red lotus flowers will enhance one's prosperity.

Saraswati Sloka

Surasura Sevita Paada Pankaja
Kare viraajita Kamaniya Pustaka
Virinchi Patni Kamalaasanastitha
Saraswati Nrutyatu Vachi me sada.

Meaning: One who is seated on a lotus, one whose lotus feet are worshipped by the Gods, one who holds a book in her hands, who is the Brahmadeva's wife, Saraswati Devi, may you be seated happily on my tongue.

Saraswati Gayatri

Om Vak Devyai cha Vidmahe
Virinchi Patnyai cha Dhimahi
Tanno Vaani Prachodayat
Om Vak Devi cha Vidmahe
Sarva Siddhicha Dhimahi
Tanno Vaani Prachodayat

Chanting the above Slokas will definitely bestow Saraswati Devi benevolent blessings upon the devotee.

Performing her puja with Saraswati Ashtottaram will bring added benefits.

Prepare a garland of white jasmines, white Arali flowers, white Nandiarvattai, marigold, Tumbaipu and garland the Devi. It is better to worship the photo of the Goddess at home. In offices, a statue of the goddess may be worshipped. If an idol is used for worship it is necessary to perform the Abhishekha for the idol regularly.

Place the books used for studies, pen, pencil, rubber, scale, Geometry box next to the photo of Saraswati while performing the puja.

Every member of the family should place one of the books of their studies, or pencil in the puja. It would be ideal for the elders to place a book of their own interest in the puja.

Apart from the above, books like the Bhagavad Gita, Vishnu Sahasranamam, and similar such spiritual books or books of sadhana, should also be placed with applying chandan and kumkum on it.

Some people have musical instruments at home such as the Veena, Violin, Tabla, Guitar, flute, Harmonium etc. which should also be placed in the puja. If there are bigger musical instruments like the Veena then one should keep it clean, apply chandan and Kumkum, cover it with a new piece of cloth and apply kumkum on it with flowers as well. If you have any jewellery of gold like a chain then the veena can be adorned with it. It is to invoke a feeling of Goddess Saraswati herself manifesting in the Veena.

Saraswati Andadi, Sakala Kalavalli songs and/or other Saraswati Stotras may be chanted in praise of the Goddess. Kings can place weapons; businessmen can place their account books, balancing scale, measuring wooden scales, Money vaults, etc at the Saraswati Puja. Workers, artisans, and craftsmen can place their regular work instruments and appliances in the puja.

Owners of factories, may place their machinery, students, their books, pen, pencils, notebooks etc. children can place their toys as well.

Music teachers may place musical instruments like the Veena, Tabla, Mrudangam, Violin, etc and perform the puja.

Sakala Vidya Saraswati Mantra
Om Hrim Shrim Vak Vageeshwari
Aim Klim Soum Mama Vak Siddham Kuru Kuru Swaha

One should chant the above mantra 1008 times every day for 21 days and complete it.

For Naivedya one should offer, milk, honey, urud Dal vada, fruits and with Dhup and Deepa perform the puja with faith and devotion. This will lead to mantra Siddhi. According to each one's spiritual development Saraswati Devi will give blessings by way of darshan, either in meditation, dream or through someone else. The one who has attained Mantra Siddhi will have Saraswati writing her aksharas on their tongue with her writing plume. From then on, all arts, limitless knowledge, poetry, and inspiration will increase. They will attain the Siddhi of speech.

May Education prosper! May Success increase! Surrender at the feet of Shri Saraswati Devi!!!